URBAN AFRICAN AMERICAN
HEALTH CARE

ERIC J. BAILEY, Ph.D.

UNIVERSITY
PRESS OF
AMERICA

Lanham • New York • London

Copyright © 1991 by

University Press of America®, Inc.

4720 Boston Way
Lanham, Maryland 20706

3 Henrietta Street
London WC2E 8LU England

Library of Congress Cataloging-in-Publication Data

Bailey, Eric J., 1958-
Urban African American health care / Eric J. Bailey.
p.   cm.
Includes bibliographical references.
1. Afro-Americans—Medical care.
2. Urban health—United States.
3. Health behavior—Michigan—Detroit—Case studies.
4. Health behavior—Texas—Houston—Case studies.   I. Title.
[DNLM: 1. Blacks. 2. Patient Acceptance of Health Care.
3. Urban Health—United States.   WA 380 B154u]
RA448.5.N4B25   1991   362.1'089'96073—dc20
DNLM/DLC for Library of Congress   91-15160 CIP

ISBN 0–8191–8277–X (paper : alk. paper)
ISBN 0–8191–8276–1 (cloth : alk. paper)

URBAN AFRICAN AMERICAN HEALTH CARE

Here is a book written by a medical anthropologist who examines the health beliefs and practices of today's urban African Americans. It is intended for health professionals, health administrators, social workers, and the general public who not only want to know more about African Americans' health care seeking pattern but also the methods to construct intervention strategies for local African American communities.

Based upon research in two major urban cities (Detroit, Michigan and Houston, Texas), this study investigates holistically the multitude of factors (cultural-historical, psychosocial and sociocultural) which influence whether or not an African American seeks health care from a variety of sources. This data is of particular importance due to the fact that African Americans' health status has continued to decline during the past several decades. This book, therefore, is the first valid investigation of today's urban African American health care.

iii

DEDICATION

For
my wife Gloria
my mother Jean
my father Roger and
all my extended family members

ACKNOWLEGEMENTS

In Acknowledging my debt to others I wish first to thank my wife Gloria Jean Bailey who has supported, encouraged, and assisted me throughout each little step of this book.

I want to thank my former dissertation committee members: Bernice Kaplan, Madeleine Leininger, Mark Weiss, and Barbara Aswad. I am also extremely grateful for the advice from Ed Sharples, Leonard Moss, and George Fathauer. The knowledge from each scholar enabled me to broaden my perspective about health care and its relationship to ethnic populations.

The following organizations also extended their cooperation and support to this study: United Health Organization, Henry Ford Hospital, Second Baptist Church, Wayne State University Graduate School, Applied Medical Anthropology Program of Wayne State University, Houston Health Department, Riverside Health Clinic, and Indiana University School of Liberal Arts.

I want to also extend my appreciation and support to Susan Sutton, Barbara Jackson, John Barlow, Bill Stuckey, Eilecee Hopkins, Marsha Neawedde, Diane Gardner, Ruth Raun, and Kokeb Teshome.

Finally, I wish to thank my parents, Roger and Jean Bailey, and my brothers, Dwight, Ronnie, Billie, and Michael for their lifelong encouragement, support, and inspiration.

PREFACE

Despite the progress made in health care during the 1980's in the United States, there continues to be a lack of cultural awareness and sensitivity to African American health problems. In fact, health problems such as hypertension, heart disease, stroke, diabetes, cancer, and infant mortality remain the major causes of death in the African American population. Moreover, a recent report investigating the disparity between African American and Anglo American health status indicates that African Americans continue to have a death rate 2.5 times HIGHER than Anglo Americans. Interestingly, this study states that before death rates among African Americans and Anglo Americans are equal, policy makers and researchers must learn more about income-related factors and identify the factors that are still unknown (Blendon et al. 1989).

Indeed, little is known about the ethnohealth and ethnocaring practices among urban African Americans. In addition, past research has also neglected how sociocultural and cultural-historical factors influence patterns of health care seeking among urban African Americans.

In 1983, as a volunteer in the Hypertension clinic of Henry Ford Hospital (Detroit, Michigan), I became intrigued about the health beliefs and health care utilization patterns among hypertensive clients. After observing staff and client ecounters for four months, I realized that a majority of clients had a different perspective form the professional staff of what constitutes "health" and what constitutes an "illness."

I also believed that African Americans' health care patterns with regards to hypertension were different than Anglo-Americans.

To research these health care issues, I designed an applied medical anthropological study. The primary purpose of this study was to produce a quantitative and qualitative analyses of Detroit African American health care patterns. Data was gathered through semi-structured and informal interviews, individual health profiles, and observations at health screening sites in the Detroit Metropolitan area. Chapter Two discusses the ethnomedical beliefs and practices of West Africans and African Americans from a cultural-historical perspective. Chapter Three examines the migration and health care strategies of Detroit African Americans from 1910 to 1980. Chapter Four discusses the research methods of the project. Chapter Five analyzes the quantitative data from the 1985 and 1986 health screenings. Chapter Six examines the qualitative data from the 1986 health screenings. Chapter Seven shows how the culturally-oriented intervention strategies developed from the Detroit study were actually implemented in a local Houston (Texas) African American community.

The secondary purpose of this study was to provide recommendations for constructing a culturally-oriented health screening program. From an applied medical anthropological perspective, culturally-oriented health care strategies are programs planned and implemented to meet the needs of the community. In particular, culturally-oriented health care strategies alert people to health care issues, inform them of the most straightforward and effective behavioral alternatives for health promotion, help them to make preventative health care choices, adopt new culture care practices, and most importantly, maintain some of their traditional ethnohealth and ethnocaring modes.

THE AUTHOR

Eric J. Bailey received his B.A. and M.A. from Miami University (Oxford, Ohio) and a Ph.D. in anthropology from Wayne State University (Detroit, Michigan). He is currently an Assistant Professor in the Anthropology Department at Indiana University (Indianapolis).His subspecialties include Medical Anthropology, Urban Anthropology and African American culture. He is also a recipient of the Minority Teaching Fellowship at Indiana University and the Thomas Rumble Fellowship at Wayne State University. He was an Instructor of Anthropology in Departments of Anthropology at the University of Houston, Wayne State University and University of Michigan, Dearborn.

Table of Contents

Chapter 1

INTRODUCTION

Currently, there are approximately 29.3 million African Americans (blacks) in the United States -- about 12.2 percent of the population. The African American population grew by 10 percent between 1980 to 1988 and 17 percent between 1970 to 1980 (United States Bureau of Census 1988 and 1980). Moreover, most African Americans (57.2%) presently live in central cities, twenty-five percent reside in suburban areas, and the remaining 17 percent in rural areas. Thus, a vast majority of African Americans (82%) are urban people. This steady increase of the African American population has not only influenced their residence patterns but in particular the type of health care they have received.

In fact, Blendon's (1989) study of 10,130 persons living in the continental United States found that even blacks above the poverty line have less access to medical care than their white counterparts. The researchers contend that ethnic-related differences in health care arrangements and lifestyle were the most significant factors in disparity between black and white health care utilization.

For example, blacks are more likely than whites to report that during their last visit their physician did not inquire sufficiently about pain, did not tell them how long it would take for prescribed medicine to work, did not explain the seriousness of the illness or injury, and did not discuss test or examination finds. In addition, fewer than three- fifths of blacks were completely satisfied with the care provided during their last hospitalization, compared with over three-fourths of whites (Blendon et al.1989). It is apparent that not only are there differences in access, but also in the perception of the care provided for blacks and whites. Blacks seem to adhere to ethnomedical beliefs and practices, and they use non-professional health care remedies more extensively than do whites.

Ironically, during the past few years, the health care field has witnessed a literal explosion of research on ethnicity and health. Sokolovsky (1985), Simic (1985), Donovan (1984), and Jackson (1981) have inspired new areas of investigation in the fields of public health, community medicine, ethnogerontology, and ethnomedicine. This ethnic revival, nevertheless, has clouded the concept of "ethnicity." As Jackson (1985: 268) states, "ethnicity is used too loosely in referring variously to racial groups, nationalistic groups and cultural groups."

In this book, "ethnicity" means peoplehood, a sense of communality or community derived from networks of family relations which have over a number of generations been the carriers of common experiences. Ethnicity, in short, means the culture of people and is thus the source of our values, attitudes, perceptions, needs, mode of expression, behaviors, and senses of identity, whether or not we are conscious of our ethnic background (Feinstein 1974:2).

Although African Americans demonstrate various cultural patterns, the African American family as a unit has a historical continuity that began not with the American experience, but in Africa long before the intrusion of Europe into that continent. The structural characteristics of the African American family include: (1) a bilateral orientation, but with the matrilateral kin often given more weight; (2) extended kin groups existing in a social environment in which primary-type relations are extended into the larger community; (3) emphasis on respect for elders; and (4) a high value placed on children and motherhood (Aschenbrenner 1973; Barnes 1981; Gutman 1976 and Hays et al. 1973).

In addition to these structural characteristics, African American families exhibit such values as: (1) a high evalua-tion of family and individual moral "strength" as a human quality; (2) an emphasis on family occasions and rituals; and a (3) strong belief in spiritualism (Aschenbrenner 1973 and Stack 1974).

With regard to health beliefs, however, little is known about the health (ethnohealth) and caring (ethnocaring) practices in urban African Americans. Studies such as Jackson (1981), Jacques (1976), LeMaile-Williams (1976), Hill (1976), Puck-ett (1969), Leininger (1985b), and Bailey (1988) illustrate that clinicians need to increase their knowledge of African American health care patterns primarily because they find it difficult to deal effectively with the needs of the African American patient.

To reiterate, utilization rates for mainstream preventative health care services are significantly different between blacks and whites. On the average, whites are twice as likely as blacks to participate in health screenings for dental, cancer, and blood pressure evaluation (Wilson 1985:263-269). In southeastern Michigan, this participation difference is quite apparent with whites using the screenings more often than blacks. During the past 20 years, a local health organization has co-sponsored a free annual multiphasic health screening in the seven county region of southeastern Michigan. Approximately, 48,000 local residents, 18 years or older, participate during the 30 day health screening each year. The percentage of African American participants, however, remains incredibly low. The fact that African Americans comprised only 6% of the 48,717 screened in 1985 and even a smaller percentage the following year (5.7%) indicates a different utilization pattern of mainstream preventative health care services among African Americans in southeastern Michigan. Thus, it is apparent that not only are there differences in utilization rates and access but also the care provided differs for African Americans and Anglo Americans along a number of dimensions; namely the adherence to health beliefs and practices and the usage of non-professional health care remedies.

African Americans' health beliefs and practices are currently a composite, containing elements from a variety of sources: European folklore, Greek classical medicine, modern scientific medicine, and particularly African folklore. These diverse threads are tied together by the tenets of fundamentalist Christianity, elements from the vodun religion of Haiti, and the added spice of sympathetic magic (Snow 1977; Jackson 1981; Jordan 1979; Crawford 1971; Jacques 1976; Baer 1985; Spector 1979; and Bailey 1988). It should be noted that this health belief system is not exclusively confined to

African Americans but also shared by segments of the Anglo American population. By analyzing the health care treatment pattern among Detroit African Americans, much can be learned about their preventive health care practices, as well as something of the preventive health care practices of other African American populations in the United States. Because the lifestyle, behavioral, and health care patterns developed by Detroit African Americans during the early 1900s to the present coincides similar patterns established in urban African American populations throughout America.

Finally, this book is not only important for all health care professionals but also for other professionals, scholars and particularly the public who sincerely care for the health and social welfare of African Americans. Moreover, it provides individuals with practical, culturally-oriented strategies to effectively mobilize and treat African Americans. This book, therefore, becomes a frame of reference that everyone can use to better understand urban African American health care.

The Study
To address the issue of African American preventive health care practices, I investigated the health care seeking behavior among 285 African Americans in the Detroit Metropolitan area. This study used hypertension as a means to examine the health care treatment pattern because more than 60 million individuals in the United States have elevated blood pressure (140/90 mmHg) or have reported being diagnosed by a

physician as having hypertension (United States Department of Health and Human Services 1986).

Hypertension is the generic term for blood pressure above defined parameters correlated with age. Currently accepted standards defining normal, borderline and high blood pressure are:

Normal: up to 138/88
Borderline: 140/90 to 158/94
High: 160/95 and higher

The probable causes of hypertension include heredity, age, sex, stress, excessive weight, high sodium intake, alcohol intake, excessive cigarette smoking and lack of exercise. Uncontrolled hypertension contributes to death and disability from stroke, coronary disease and kidney failure. (Comprehensive Health Planning Council of Southeastern Michigan 1979:v-25).

The prevalence rate of hypertension among blacks (38.2%) is still substantially higher than among whites (28.2%). African Americans, for example, show rates of moderate hypertension that are two times that of Whites, and rates of severe hypertension that are three times greater. This difference in relative frequency is more marked in African American males, among whom the rate of severe elevations (2.2%) is over four times greater than in white males (0.5%). Moreover, African American females show the highest prevalence of isolated systolic hypertension (2.4%), which is predominantly seen in the elderly (National High Blood Pressure Education Program Coordinating Committee 1985). A disheartening aspect of this health problem in African Americans and other high risk groups is that adherence to an effective treatment regimen and/or an increased utilization of health screenings can prevent approximately 50% of the deaths associated with hypertension.

The most perplexing attribute of essential hypertension is that there are usually no symptoms associated with it -- it is asymptomatic. According to hypertension clinicians, a person cannot tell what his/her blood pressure is by how he/she feels. The only way to know one's pressure is to have it measured.

At the time of measurement, the hypertension clinician should discuss the following items with the patient: (a) the numerical blood pressure value; (b) the need for periodic remeasurement; and (c) available antihypertensive treatment including specific drugs and results. In addition, with those individuals whose pressures are elevated, the clinician should inquire about: (a) previous treatment for hypertension; (b) the desirability of hypertension control; and (c) the potential dangers of uncontrolled hypertension.

However, most people are unaccustomed of thinking about illness in asymptomatic terms because symptoms provide the starting point for speculations about illness. Garro (1988), Dressler (1982), and Blumhagen (1982) contend that individuals develop "common sense models" or "cultural definitions" of hypertension in an attempt to treat the disease. Such symptoms as headaches, dizziness, tiredness, flushing sensations, and nervousness or anxiety are commonly associated with hypertension. These symptoms, therefore, help to formulate the individual's "cultural definition" of hypertension.

Focus of Study

To assess the factors which affect blood pressure level and health care seeking pattern, the following hypotheses were tested:

1. Sociodemographic and psychosocial factors significantly influence blood pressure levels.

2. As national health statistics indicate, African Americans will exhibit higher blood pressure levels than Anglo Americans.

3. African Americans will demonstrate an alternative health care seeking pattern to Anglo Americans.

4. Sociocultural and cultural-historical factors significantly influence African Americans utilization of mainstream health screening facilities.

5. African Americans health (ethnomedical) beliefs in particular with regard to hypertension significantly influence their pattern of health care seeking.

Utilizing the United Health Organization's facilities for interviewing, I conducted a two-phase study during the operation of the 1985 and 1986 Project Health-O-Rama health screenings. In 1985, I interviewed 82 African Americans and 96 Anglo Americans at seven sites in the Detroit

Metropolitan area. These sites included community health centers, churches, and malls. The instruments used in this 1985 sample were Becker's Health Belief Questionnaire (1977) and Spielberger's State Anxiety Inventory (1970) with slight modifications made by the researcher. Standard parametric statistics tested the health belief indices, anxiety scores, and sociodemographic variables of the general informants. The initial research at the 1986 health screenings paralleled the methods used in 1985. Additionally, the 1986 study included more data focusing on individual health profiles. The sample consisted of 203 African Americans (semi-structured interviews and individual health profiles) and 82 Anglo Americans (semi-structured interviews). The quantitative data were analyzed separately and later integrated with the qualitative ethnographic data to construct a holistic analyses of African Americans' health care seeking pattern.

The four major goals of this study were as follows:

1. Examine the sociodemographic and psychosocial factors which affect blood pressure level.

2. Investigate the health beliefs and preventive health care practices of African Americans.

3. Determine how African Americans' health (ethnomedical) beliefs in particular with regard to hypertension influence their pattern of health care seeking.

4. Provide recommendations for constructing a culturally-oriented health screening program.

To assess whether the recommendations of the Detroit study were truly effective, this medical anthropologist collaborated with local health officials and residents in Houston, Texas (1989) to design a community health screening program. Chapter 7 discusses entirely the development, the design, and the implementation of a culturally-oriented community health screening program for a local African American population.

The following section highlights the social and health care dynamics of southeastern Michigan for the purpose of understanding the health care patterns of Detroit African Americans.

SOUTHEASTERN MICHIGAN

Identity

African Americans are primarily descendants of West African people who share a common history, place of origin, language, food preferences, health beliefs, and values that engender a sense of exclusiveness and self-awareness of being a member of this ethnic group. Despite the distinctive qualities of each West African tribe, African Americans held to a set of cultural beliefs and patterns which were common among West African people. Several researchers, for instance, contend that West African traits such as an extended family network, a strong belief in spiritualism, and an admiration of older adults, are still exemplified in varying degrees among African Americans regardless of regional or social class variations (Staples 1981; Crosby et al. 1981; Franklin and Moss 1988; Hines and Boyd-Franklin 1982; Harding 1981; Berry 1982; and Pinderhughes 1982).

African Americans' cultural beliefs and patterns, have been modified by acculturation and assimilation to mainstream North American society over the centuries. Currently, African Americans living in Northern parts of the United States tend to have more egalitarian relationships between parents and children and between men and women than the traditional patterns of southern families. Independence and autonomy orientation have replaced strict adherence to authority figures. Nevertheless, there are two cultural traits that distinguish African Americans from other immigrant groups in the United States: (1) they were composed of many different tribes, each with its own languages, cultures, and traditions; and (2) they came in bondage (Billingsley 1968).

Setting

The city of Detroit is located in the seven-county region of southeastern Michigan. Within this geographically diverse region are urban, suburban, and rural subareas as well as many cultural and ethnic groups (Greater Detroit Area Health Council 1983). Figure 1 and Tables 1.1 and 1.2 show the location of the seven counties in Michigan and Wayne County's population distribution by ethnicity. In 1980, the population of southeastern Michigan was 4,482,782. The population had grown by 13% during the 1960-1970 period but had experienced a one percent decline in the following

MICHIGAN (LOWER PENINSULA)

FIGURE 1
SOUTHEASTERN MICHIGAN COUNTIES

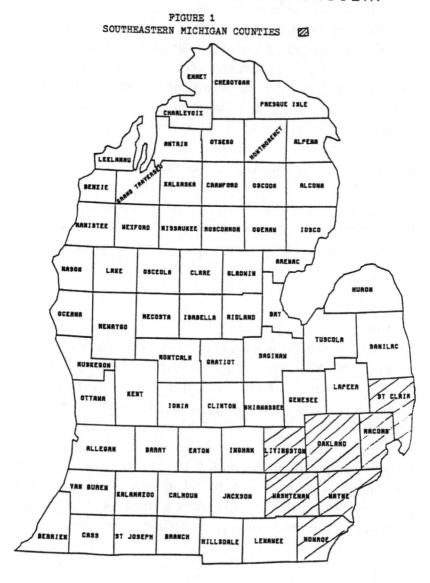

Table 1.1:   Population Distribution by Ethnicity - 1970 & 1980

Wayne County

	Black		Spanish Origin	
	No.	%	No.	%
1970	721,072	27.04	41,195	1.54
1980	829,868	35.70	46,301	1.99

Table 1.2:   Population Distribution by Ethnicity - 1970 & 1980

Wayne County

American Indian		Asian Origin		All Other	
No.	%	No.	%	N	%
1970					
4,419	.16	6,490	.24	6,270	.23
1980					
6,667	.29	15,164	.65	28,132	1.21

Comprehensive Health Planning of S.E. MI 1981)

ten years. This one percent decline translates to a net out-migration of 400,000 people during the 1970-1980 decade. Within the City of Detroit (Wayne County), the population declined from 40% of the regional total in 1960 to 26% of the total in 1980. The redistribution of the population caused increases in Livingston, St. Clair, Monroe, and Washtenaw

Counties and in the "outer" suburbs of Wayne, Oakland, and Macomb counties.

During the 1980s, Detroit's population continued to decline. In 1987, census data reported 1,217,000 in the city of Detroit, down 60,000 from 1980. The decline of Detroit's population reflects the continual out-migration of city residents to the suburbs. In addition, this populational trend dramatically affected the age, sex, and racial composition of southeastern Michigan.

From 1960 to 1980, the proportion of the population in southeastern Michigan over 65 increased from 7.2 to 9.4 percent, while the age cohort 0-14 years of age decreased by 300,000 individuals (or 9.3 percent). The proportions of people over 65 increased most markedly in Macomb and Oakland counties (by 3.4%) and in Wayne County (by 2.4%). By 1980, approximately 11.7% of the population of the City of Detroit was 65 years or older, as compared with only 6.4% in the older age category in Washtenaw County.

The southeastern Michigan's proportion of non-white residents grew from 14.0 to 21.7 percent with the most dramatic change in the City of Detroit where the racial turnover changed from 70.8% white in 1960 to 65.6% non-white in 1980. Tables 1.3 - 1.8 show the 1980 estimated numbers and percentages of the city's non-white and white distribution (see appendix). As of 1990, Detroit's African American population comprised 67% of the total population. Substantial increases in the proportions of non-whites also occurred in Washtenaw and Oakland Counties during the 1970-1980 decade. Moreover, the proportions of females in the region's population increased from 50.6 to 51.5 percent. In the City of Detroit, the female percentage is 52.7 (Greater Detroit Area Health Council 1983).

Economic Conditions
The state of Michigan has always been a leader in industrial manufacturing with much of the production centered in the Detroit metropolitan area. Over the years, however, there has been a shift away from the region's earlier concentration of manufacturing. While the region's total number of jobs increased from 1970 to 1980, the number of manufacturing jobs declined 20 percent. The loss of manufacturing jobs caused the unemployment rate to increase steadily.

By 1980, the unemployment rate in the Detroit Metropolitan area reached 14% as a result of declining car sales and the general recessionary economy. The rippling effect of the high unemployment rates resulted in 16.4% (483,258 persons) of Wayne County families living below the U.S. poverty guideline (Comprehensive Health Planning Council of S.E. Michigan 1981). Moreover, the percentages of families living in poverty among female headed households with children and heads of household 65 years or older were 46% and 16% (Michigan Metropolitan Information Center 1983). Such unemployment trends coupled with the percentage of persons 25 and over who do not have a high school education (38% in Wayne County), and other sociodemographic statistics (Wayne County's median family income - $22,000 and Public Assistant Recipients - 20.7%), had a direct impact on the region's health care delivery system and the health status of its citizen.

Health Care Delivery System and Health Status

Health Resources

In southeastern Michigan, hospitals range in size from those of less than 50 beds to some with more than one thousand beds. Some are of limited purpose scope whereas others offer varying levels of comprehensiveness in medicine, surgery, obstetrics, pediatrics, psychiatry, rehabilitation, the several subspecialties, supplementary services, education, research, and out-of-hospital services (Greater Detroit Area Council 1983:36).

Over the last two decades, a clear trend toward fewer, larger, and more fully utilized hospitals has developed in southeastern Michigan. For example, the number of general acute care hospitals serving southeastern Michigan declined 29 percent from 108 to 77 facilities. The largest decrease occurred in Detroit by 1980 with 37 specialty and acute care hospitals closed with a loss of 1,700 beds during the last twenty years.

In the area of outpatient services, hospitals in central Detroit also experienced a decline of approximately 10 percent per year in both emergency room and outpatient clinic visits between 1980 and 1982 after a slight increase between 1979 and 1980. In contrast, the number of outpatient clinic visits in the entire region experienced a gradual increase since 1979 which is at least partially explained by the development of decentralized outpatient facilities outside of central Detroit (Reilly 1983:46).

Health Personnel Resources

Of those who actually deliver health care, approximately 50% of the 100,000 health workers in southeastern Michigan worked in professional and technical capacities. Southeastern Michigan has an estimated 9,000 physicians in active practice, of whom 84% had "allopathic" and 16% had osteopathic education. Half of the osteopathic physicians and 40% of the allopathic physicians delivered primary care (family practice, general practice, OB-GYN, internal medicine, or pediatrics).

The ratio of physician to population increased by 45.5 percent since 1960 (from 1.32 to 1.92 per 1,000 population) and is expected to increase another 27 percent (to 2.44) by 1990. This rate of increase was slightly higher than state and national trends. Specifically, there is currently one physician for every 522 people in this seven-county region; and it is expected that there will be one physician for every 410 people in the region by 1990 (Greater Detroit Area Council 1983:38).

The largest health profession in southeastern Michigan is nursing which has more than 22,000 actively practicing professionals. Currently, the ratio of practicing to licensed nurses is relatively high. The proportion of working licensed nurses increased during the 1960s and 1970s from approximately 65 percent to 80 percent. There is concern, however, that the nursing shortage during the 1980s may continue in the 1990s (Greater Detroit Area Health Council 1983:39).

Other prominent health care providers include physician assistants, nurse practitioners, clinical nurse specialists, and nurse clinicians. If southeastern Michigan has already an abundance of physicians, it is projected that economic competition will make it very difficult for nurse practitioners, physician assistants, and other health care providers to find security in this health care job market (Greater Detroit Area Health Council 1983:39).

Utilization of Services

Between 1974 and 1982, the number of patients per 1,000 population admitted to the southeastern Michigan hospitals increased slightly (from 150.8/1,000 to 160.1/1,000). The number of patient days per 1,000 population, however declined slightly (from 1,372.6/1,000 to 1,355.4/1,000). Nevertheless, the use of hospital services increased by age category, with people 65 and over using 4.597 patient days per 1,000 people in this age category -- or about four times as much as people under age 65. In fact, the 1980 patient day use rate in southeastern Michigan was higher than state and national rates in every age category except the 0-14 age group.

Persons who were members of Health Maintenance Organizations (HMOs) also exhibited a different health care utilization pattern than did non-members. The southeastern Michigan HMO enrolles, who represented about five percent of the private insurance market, used hospitals at the rate of 500 days per thousand compared to non-members rate of 1,355 days per thousand. This relatively high rate among HMO enrolles was primarily because: (1) a high proportion of young participants (usually not typical HMO members) and (2) visiting nursing services increased (Greater Detroit Area Health Council 1983:46).

Health Care Costs

Approximately $6 billion was spent on health care in southeastern Michigan during 1981. Estimated per capita expenditures for all health services within the region was $1,282. This was about 25 percent higher than the national cost per capita that year.

Southeastern Michigan health care expenditures have historically been higher than the averages of most metropolitan areas and of the nation as a whole (Greater Detroit Area Health Council 1983). In 1980, for example, average cost per stay ($3,308) and average cost per day ($414) were higher than the national average ($1,851 stay; $245 cost per day). The reasons for the escalated health care costs involved such factors as the state of the economy, population characteristics, and regulatory programs (Greater Detroit Area Health Council 1983:111).

Causes of Death

The causes of death among southeastern Michigan residents were similar to the national pattern: (1) heart disease, (2) cancer, (3) cerebrovascular disease, and (4) accidents. Table 1.9 shows the major causes of death in the State and Wayne County (see appendix). The percentage of deaths from heart disease was approximately 40% for all seven counties except Washtenaw (35%). Non-disease causes of death showed considerable variation from county to county, with motor vehicle accidents being highest in Livingston County; suicides highest in Washtenaw County, and homicides most common in Wayne County. The death rates for Wayne County residents far exceed those in other southeastern counties. These health statistics as well as the health care delivery statistics indicate that Detroit residents were definitely in need of health care and social services.

CONCLUSION

This brief overview of the health care delivery system and the sociodemographic characteristics associated with southeastern Michigan residents suggests that a number of new health care and economic programs need to be implemented throughout this region. According to the 1985 Report of the Secretary Task Force of the Department of Health and Human Services on Blacks & Minority Health Issues and the 1987 National Health Epidemiological Survey, research on the relationship between health beliefs and health care seeking behavior may assist in explaining the patterns of health care for some ethnic populations. Moreover, such research would provide a frame of reference that health professionals could use to better understand the social ills and special problems among ethnic populations (LeMaile-Williams 1976). This research was therefore designed for health care professionals, public health administrators, and the general public who are concerned with the biological, psychological, sociological, and culturological well-being of African Americans in today's urban society.

Chapter 2

URBAN AFRICAN AMERICAN HEALTH CARE

INTRODUCTION

The study of how members of different cultures think about disease and organize themselves toward medical treatment and the social organization of treatment itself is referred to as ethnomedicine (Fabrega 1975:969). Ethnomedical studies have researched such topics as culturally unique disorders like susto (soul loss) among Hispanics (Rubel 1977), the adaptive role of the barefoot healers of China (New and New 1977), the relationship between health and harmony in the beliefs of Navajo (Adair and Deuschle 1977) and the etiological beliefs of middle-income Anglo Americans (Chino and Vollweiler 1986). In general, ethnomedical studies focus upon a culture's disease classification, the ethnomedical therapy, and the cultural aspects of ethnomedicine (Lieban 1977). This chapter discusses the preceding three issues of ethnomedicine in reference to the development of African American health beliefs and practices with particular emphasis concerning the health care seeking process among African Americans.

WEST AFRICAN ETHNOMEDICAL BELIEFS

Although current African American ethnomedical beliefs and practices have diverse sources, much of the system derives from the traditional health beliefs of West African cultures. In West African cultures, life was viewed as a process rather than as a state, and the nature of a person was viewed in terms of energy force rather than of matter. (Harvey 1988, Jacques 1976, Mbiti 1975, Puckett 1969, Spector 1979). Moreover, all things, whether living or dead, were believed to influenced each other. One had the power, therefore, to influence one's destiny and that of others through the use of behavior as well as through knowledge of the person and the world (Spector 1979:231). Maintaining one's health meant harmony with nature, whereas illness was a state of disharmony. Hence, traditional West African ethnomedical beliefs perceived health as a dynamic process of the mind, body, and spirit (Jacques 1976:116).

Illness was attributed to naturalistic and personalistic causative agents. West Africans related the disruption of the ecosystem, such as weather changes, with occurrence of minor illnesses. Minor complaints like stomach upsets, headaches, cuts, and skin ulcers thus were normally treated with herbs and other medicines generally known to each community (Mbiti 1975 and Goodson 1987).

Serious or severe illnesses, however, were primarily attributed to personalistic agents such as demons and evil spirits. These spirits were generally believed to act on their own accord. Ethnomedical treatment involved removing the spiritual entity from the ill person's body. Medicine men, herbalists, diviners, mediums, seers, priests, and even rulers conducted this ritual (Mbiti 1975:170, Puckett 1969).

These traditional healers (both men and women) used religious and spiritual means to find out the cause of disease, and to uncover the individual responsible for sending it. Traditional healers utilized religious rituals, herbs and roots, and the observance of certain prohibitions or directions to cure individuals (Mbiti 1975). To assure the sick person that the illness would not recur, traditional healers suggested that maintaining religious steps and observances could act as preventive measures.

When traditional healers could not cure the individual, a direct appeal to God was the final answer. Since native West Africans believed that God is the ultimate source of all medicines, it was logical to by-pass human dealers in medicine and appeal to God directly for his intervention (Mbiti 1975:174). Finally, West African ethnomedical beliefs concerning the use of traditional medicines generates confidence and a sense of security among individuals who have little control over the forces of human nature. Mbiti (1975) summarizes the following about West African ethnomedicine:

"Whether traditional medicines function in every case or not need not matter very much. It is the belief in the efficacy of such medicine which inspires hope in the sick, confidence in the the hunter and businessman, courage in the sufferer and the traveller, and a sense of security in the many who feel that they are surrounded by mystical and physical enemies. This in itself is a valuable benefit gained from the belief in medicine as West African peoples understand and apply it." (Mbiti 1975:174)

AFRICAN AMERICAN ETHNOMEDICAL BELIEFS

As early as the 1500s and 1600s, West Africans were forcibly transported to South America, the Carribean, and North America. In the process of adapting to the new environments, West Africans merged their cultural traditions with European and Native American traditions.

African Americans nevertheless retained many of the preventive and treatment practices associated with indigenous West African cultures primarily because these methods were perceived to be most useful. Jacques (1976), Jordan (1975), Jackson (1985), Baer (1985), Spector (1979), Goodson (1987), Mbiti (1975), Puckett (1969), Harvey (1988), Tinling (1967), and Tallant (1990) all contend that African Americans continued to utilize folk and herbal medical practices as a result of the communication difficulties with Europeans and the fear of European physicians. Traditional West African ethnomedical beliefs and practices were handed down and maintained among various African American populations throughout North America (Spector 1979:232).

According to Goodson (1987), such medicinal plants as *Chenopodium ambrosioides* (Jerusalem oak), *Eupatorium perfoliatum* (boneset), *Aristolochia serpentia* (one of the snake roots), and *Podophyllum peltatum* (May apple) were used extensively among transplanted Africans for preventing and curing diseases. Oral histories of former slave women from all over the South contained frequent and sometimes elaborate descriptions of the wide variety of plants which constituted the material base from which the slave medical practice operated (Goodson 1987:200).

Female African American slave doctors, for example, used drugs derived from plants to prevent and cure worms, malaria, croup, pneumonia, colds, teething, and measles. Sometimes, they used the root, at other times, they selected the leaf, bark, fruit or gum resin to boil into a tea or make into a poultice or wear in a bag around the neck (Goodson 1987:200).Not only did African American slave doctors have this medical botanical knowledge of plants, but also many other slaves knew how to diagnose and how to treat illnesses. In fact,a number of medicine chests have been discovered filled with the popular preparations of the day: calomel, blue mass pills, castor oil, ipecac, tartar emetic, and various tinctures (Ewell 1813).

During the 1700s and 1800s in the United States, African American ethnomedical beliefs and practices continued to show similarities with the West Africans' and Haitians' religion, "Voodoo" or "Vodoun" (Tallant 1990). As a form of religion, Voodoo is a complex of African belief and ritual governing in large measure the religious life of the African natives (Herskovits 1937:139). Harvey (1988) states that "as a belief system which combined historical conceptions with practices that were acceptable in a hostile social environment, Voodoo is a striking example of a cultural adaptive mechanism used by members of an oppressed group as a survival technique." The African American form of Voodoo medicine consisted of three major components.

The first is the mystic component which deals with the supernatural such as spells and spirits. The second component is that part of voodoo which deals with psychological support of the individual, and the third part is herbal and folk medicine. African American voodoo prospered particularly in the south primarily because it filled a void left by inaccess and denial of medical care by traditional American physicians (Jordan 1979:38). Thus, African American ethnomedical beliefs and practices merged with elements from the Voodoo religion of Haiti and Africa in an effort to treat the individual biologically and spiritually.

As more African Americans migrated to Northern cities during the mid 1800s and early 1900s, they brought a repertoire of health care beliefs and practices. African American ethnomedical beliefs and practices, thus, became a composite, containing elements from a variety of sources: European folklore, Greek classical medicine, modern scientific medicine, Vodun religion, Christianity, and particularly African folklore (Hill 1976). With such a mixture of health belief systems, it is no wonder why African American ethnomedical beliefs and practices are currently shared by all segments of the American population.

AFRICAN AMERICAN HEALTH CARE SEEKING BE-HAVIOR

In an effort to understand today's African American health care practices, we must review their process of seeking health care. This investigation is critically important because we not only learn much information about their health care practices but also the health care practices of other ethnic groups in the United States.

Health care seeking behavior is a concept which describes the events that take place when a person is sick. This behavioral pattern includes steps taken by an individual who perceives a need for help as he or she attempts to solve a health problem (Chrisman 1977:353). These steps are conceptually differentiated as elements in the health care seeking process: (1) symptom definition (2) illness-related shifts in role behavior, (3) lay consultation and referral, (4) treatment actions, and (5) adherence (Chrisman 1977:353). Figure 2 illustrates a schematic depiction of the health care seeking elements and the major directions of influence.

An individual does not necessarily follow the sequential format of the health care seeking process, but he/she usually identifies with the importance and value each element conveys within its sociocultural setting. If a sick person interacts with others at some point during the illness, for example, he may be simultaneously receiving aid in categorizing symptoms, bargaining for the legitimacy of avoiding role obligations, receiving support or information from peers and family members, and obtaining treatment from peers and family members, and obtaining treatment or practitioner suggestions (Chrisman 1977). Hence, the health care seeking model enables investigators to explicitly link sociocultural factors to individual behavior during sickness.

Figure 2.1   HEALTH SEEKING PROCESS

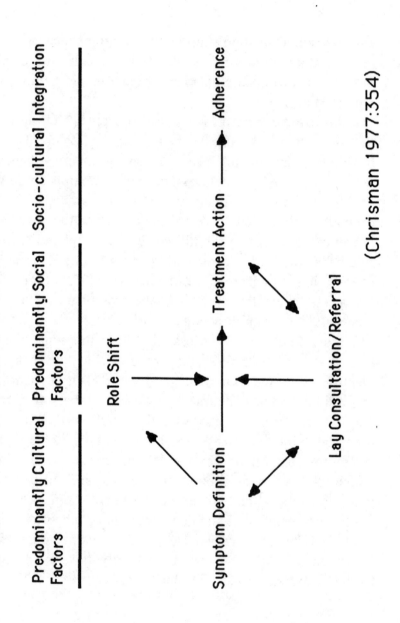

(Chrisman 1977:354)

Components of the Health Care Seeking Process

Symptom Definition

According to the health care seeking model, an individual's symptom definition develops when the degree of discomfort becomes noticeable and acknowledgeable by his/her cultural group. If the illness receives a 'cultural stamp', then, a health care action follows (Chrisman 1977). While African Americans are highly observant and attentive to perceived symptoms, sociocultural and psychosocial factors may prevent personal and public recognition of such discomforts.

For example, although there is a distinction between good and poor health, African Americans' perception of what constitutes 'healthy' encompasses a relatively high tolerance of discomforts from symptoms (Jackson 1981). Studies have shown that African Americans often ignore minor discomforts as backaches, upset stomach, or headaches until they reach such proportions that they interfere with the business of living (Jackson 1981). In fact, African Americans, particularly the elderly, often perceive their health status in "poorer" condition than Anglo Americans (Manuel 1986). Furthermore, since one's self-esteem, sanity, and survival are at risk, in a state of health (good or bad), one becomes adaptive, flexible, alert, and able to use a wide range of strategies effectively to endure and reach his/her optimal potential. In other words, until the degree of discomfort impairs daily activities or acknowledged by the individual's sociocultural network, seeking health care, particularly from mainstream health care facilities, is not warranted.

Since "illness" is physically, socially, emotionally, spiritually and/or culturally defined, African Americans perceive this stage as a loss or self, a sense of disharmony with one's soul, or being "the only one," "lost," and lacking communion with others (Jacques 1976:121 and Leininger 1985). The cause of one's illness is classified as either naturalistic or personalistic.

As stated earlier in this chapter, naturalistic agents identify what caused an illness, whereas personalistic agents recognize who caused the illness (Chino and Volleweiler 1986). Such impersonal agents as inadequate rest, poor nutrition, and germs cause illnesses. The etiology of illnesses fall into three general categories: environmental hazards, divine punishment, and impaired sociocultural relationships.

In some cases, serious and life-threatening illnesses are perceived to be sent by God (personalistic agent) as punishment for sin (Snow 1974 and Hill 1976). Many African Americans, for example, who suspect a terminal illness may delay medical diagnosis. During this delay and/or denial period, many African Americans turn to powers considered greater than themselves to fathom the reason for the disease; thereby accepting terminal illness as "God's will" and nothing more can be done.

In summary, the symptom definition of illness among African Americans is highly contingent upon a multitude of factors. Since Man is viewed as a biopsychosocial, spiritual, and cultural being, African Americans strive to maintain harmony with himself/herself and the universe by expanding his/her definition of what constitutes "healthy;" contrarily reducing his acknowledgement of what may be defined

physiologically as an "illness." From this perspective one's
illness can be perceived as "ill-at-ease -- a state of dis-ease"
without being functionally incapacitated (Jacques 1976:121).
This process relates to the second stage of the health care
seeking model - illness-related shifts in role behavior.

Illness-Related Shifts in Role Behavior

Since all cultural and ethnic groups associate modified rights
and obligations with the so-called "sick role," often the ill
person among African Americans cannot readily adopt this
role behavior. Some African Americans may even have am-
bivalent feelings of sick relatives or friends because they are
relieved of family duties. This happens frequently to African
American females who are expected to remain well despite
varing socioeconomic and cultural constraints in order to care
for the family.

Nevertheless, when family members are perceived as being
ill and incapable of carrying out their role responsibilites,
they are usually relieved of these duties (Jackson 1981:88). In
fact, assistance from kin (particularly adult children) and non-
kin members provides substantial emotional and physical
caring for the ill person (Leininger 1985 and U.S. Department
of Health and Human Services 1986).

The impaired African American elderly receive particularly
special attention. Studies have shown that the African
American elderly generally receive more supportive services
from both formal and informal support systems than did
Anglo American elderly (Jackson 1981 and Mindel et al.

1981). Furthermore, not only did African Americans receive more support quantitatively than Anglo Americans but also "qualitatively" from various sources within the community (Mindel et al. 1981). The ill person and also the caregiver thus cooperate in a "bargaining" process for the purpose of restoring the health and function of the sick person.

Lay Consultation and Referral

The patterns of lay consultation and referral among African Americans illustrate how the extensive sociocultural network influences their health care seeking pattern. Not surprisingly, the wife/mother/grandmother is customarily expected to monitor the symptoms and direct the course of action of the ill person. If the female has an ill elderly parent, she also cares for him/her. In two-parent households, nonetheless, both spouses participate in joint decisions about medical treatment for their offspring and each other (Jackson 1981:89).

Lay consultation and referral outside the household is likely to derive initially from friends and/or relatives as opposed to health care professionals. Sokolovsky (1985) found that African Americans were more likely to discuss their illness with extended family members and friends than Anglo Americans. In fact, African American womens' lay consultation network exhibited a greater variety and depth of instrumental and emotional types of support than Anglo Americans. The health care implication this difference makes is that the African American women's sociocultural network tends to be highly adaptable in dealing with acute medical, psychological, and other daily living crises (Sokolovsky 1985:10).

In conclusion, the major reasons why African Americans utilize extensively their informal lay sociocultural network for health care problems are: (1) the reciprocal give-and-take relationships between the individual and family, friends, neighbors, or acquaintances can act as a buffer between the individual and the stressful situation; (2) that these sources can alleviate the stress by helping the person instrumentally or by helping the person psychologically better cope with the situation; and (3) the opportunity for everyone to be involved in the healing process.

Treatment Actions

The types and sources of treatment actions among African Americans are likely to vary according to class, region of the United States, and degree of assimilation to mainstream society. In the United States, most ethnic groups have the option of selecting from a variety of sources: (1) formal health professionals; (2) licensed health practitioners; (3) alternative or native health practitioners; (4) lay consultation; and (5) self. As indicated in the preceding subheading, lay consultation is an important treatment option for African Americans.

The lay informal sociocultural network often employ a variety of home remedies or patent medicine. Spector (1979) documents a few home remedies practiced among African Americans.

1. Numerous types of poultices are employed to fight infection and inflammation. The poultices are placed on the part of the body that is painful and/or infected, in order to draw out the cause of the affliction.

2. A method for treating colds is with hot lemon water with honey.

3. When congestion is present in the chest and the person is coughing, he can be wrapped with warm flannel after his chest is rubbed with hot camphorated oil.
   (Spector 1979:237)

Regardless of the type of home remedy or patent medicine used by the individual, self-prescribed home medications are generally taken prior to medical consultations and continued after consultation with prescribed medications without the physician's knowledge.

The physician may not be informed of another source of treatment action which is common among African Americans - the use of the alternative or native health practitioner. There are primarily four types of alternative health practitioners serving the African American community: (1) independent generalist, (2) independent specialist, (3) cultic generalist, and (4) cultic specialist (Baer 1985:327). The independent practitioner operates as an individual or is affiliated with some sort of occult supply store, either as the owner, an employee, or someone who rents office space. In reference to the cultic practitioner, he/she is affiliated with a religious group and practices in both public and private settings. The

multiplicity of African American alternative health practitioners today stems from the role adaptability of traditional
African healers of the past.

   In fact, the ethnohealing practices of African American alternative health practitioners today are quite similar to those
of West African folk healers. For instance, one type of
African American alternative health practitioner, the neighborhood prophet/Old lady, does not dispense medicine, but
merely advises clients of concocting herbal medicines. Rather
than selling or giving a herbal remedy, the Old Lady tells the
client to use it in varying proportions to treat the perceived
illness. In addition, she also gives advice for various emotional, personal, and domestic problems. She does not receive
monetary gifts for her service only gifts of food or expression
of gratitude (Jordan 1979:38). The neighborhood prophet/Old
Lady treats the individual's mind, body, and spirit in an attempt to return the individual to harmony with nature.

   African Americans tend to consult an alternative health
practitioner primarily because of: (1) their attempt to cope
with health problems within the context of one's resources
and sociocultural environment; (2) their belief that alternative
health practitioners have some control over the forces that
cause anomalies in a person's life, whereas westernized medical physicians cannot heal certain cases of illness and misfortune and (3) lower monetary expense associated with such
treatments (Cockerham 1986:88 and Hill 1976:14).

Adherence

The final step of the health care seeking process, adherence, refers to the degree to which the sick person acts upon the treatment advice. The adherence of African Americans to traditional remedies as well as the difficulty some African American patients have in understanding the biomedical presentation of physicians and to participate actively in the discussion of their illness affect not only the quality of care but also the adherence to prescribed treatment regimens.

The fact that 50 percent of all patients fail in adhering to prescribed treatment regimen, regardless of race, remains a major issue for most health care professionals (Morisky 1986). This high rate of nonadherence, especially among African Americans, can substantially be reduced by simply implementing the following measures:

1. Gain knowledge of African American health beliefs and practices.

2. Respect the fact that although cultural beliefs in the value of folk therapies may run counter to the scientific medical systems, they have survived through several generations and may be quite effective in helping African American clients. Changing deeply rooted health beliefs through ridicule and skepticism not only may fail but may also alienate the African American patient.

3. Support the extended family and social network of African Americans, as it is vital to their health and survival.

Implementing these practical measures should improve adherence as well as the social bond with many African American patients.

CONCLUSION

This review of the health care seeking process in the context of African American culture reflects a broader understanding of the factors which influence their health care action. Moreover, the cultural-historical analysis of African American health care beliefs and practices gave the reader a special insight regarding the ethnic and sociocultural bond an individual may develop toward his/her health beliefs and practices.

The persistence of traditional African American health beliefs and practices provides a meaningful alternative to allopathic medicine for many African Americans because of its role in maintaining a sense of ethnic identity. It also indicates a pattern of adaptation to social and economic conditions both within the African American community and in the larger society. Once we recognize, understand and decide to work within the framework of the multitude of factors that influences African American health care practices, increased adherence to such health care issues as hypertension, cancer, and prenatal treatment programs can finally be improved.

Chapter 3

CULTURAL HISTORICAL BACKGROUND OF DETROIT AFRICAN AMERICANS

INTRODUCTION

Before examining the health care beliefs and practices of Detroit African Americans, a cultural-historical review of the African American migration and acculturation provides an opportunity to investigate the adaptability of this ethnic group in relationship to the region's economic, social, political, and health care systems. The lifestyle and behavior patterns acquired by Detroit African Americans during the early 1900s to the mid 1950s coincided with similar patterns established in urban African American populations throughout the Northern and Western regions of the United States. Often African American migrants entered dramatically different environments which varied from their home locales in climate, foods, available work and leisure activities, housing and sanitation facilities, and in expected cultural behaviors and social relations, crowded housing, language differences, varying ethnic prejudices etc., but even in clothing, patterns of bodily movement and access to help when needed (Kaplan 1988:221). This chapter will highlight not only the social and health conditions of each period, but will also show how the adaptive strategies, particularly the ethnomedical and mainstream

41

health care utilization patterns, are still quite apparent among today's Detroit African Americans.

AFRICAN AMERICANS: 1910 - 1965

The migration of African Americans out of the rural South from 1910 to 1930 took on the aspect of a mass movement. This great migration of African Americans into northern urban areas became one of the most significant events in the history of African Americans in the 20th century (Palmer 1967). Estimates suggests that over one million African Americans (ten percent) fled the South for Northern communities (Marks 1985). In fact, 73 percent of the Northern African Americans could be found in ten of the Northern urban centers (Palmer 1967:53).

According to Marks (1985), a number of push-pull factors significantly influenced the Southern African Americans' migratory pattern to the North. Pushed-out of the South because of the boll weevil, flooding, disenfranchisment, and the effect of the Jim Crow act, African American migrants were at the same time pulled North by increased demand for their labor.

By 1915, the North desperately needed labor. With the war in Europe, the arrival of foreign immigrants gradually dwindled to one-fourth (110,618) of its 1914 total. Northern industrial employers were obliged to find a substitute labor source. Recognizing their predicament, the Northern industrial employers implemented a decisive plan of action. By slowly curtailing the discriminatory employment practices against Northern African Americans and increasingly recruiting Southern African Americans, the Northern industries filled a void.

African Americans felt that the new labor markets in the North would provide them social, economic, and political freedom which did not exist in the South. For example, wages in the South were low and opportunities for African Americans were limited. Marks (1985) noted that for those in non-agricultural work, wages ranged from about $1.25 a day for laborers to $3.00 a day for artisans. While those in agriculture earned about $.75 per day, the majority received no wages at all, working instead for payments in kind. Considering that 80 percent of Southern African Americans lived in rural areas and were predominantly agricultural workers, average wages in the South were only about three-fourths of those in the Northern urban areas (Marks 1985:152).

Migrants often heard about the wages and opportunities in the North from labor recruiters. These people were employees of Northern companies who traveled extensively in Southern cities bringing word of employment. At the beginning of the great migration, labor recruiters purchased train "passes" for workers and also cooperated with the local African American press to glamorize conditions in the North. Marks (1985) claims that the large volume of African American migrants was directly attributable to labor recruiters.

The devasting impact of the boll weevil also brought African American laborers to the North. The boll weevil, an insect that fed on cotton bolls, entered Texas in 1898 and migrated in a state-by-state march destroying all cotton in its path. This infestation threw hundreds of thousands of agricultural laborers off the land, out of rural areas and into Southern cities; thereby causing increased competition for the limited city jobs. As unemployment continued to rise, Southern African Americans were forced to find an alternative means of survival -- to migrate North.

Although the increased employment opportunities and higher wages in the North were significant inducements to migrants, other advantages existed. The possibility of getting a good education, safety from racial violence and lynchings, and the fact that African Americans could vote and hold office in the North was a strong factor to many. Thus, a number of major factors influenced African American families (including extended family members) to migrate Northward for the urban enclaves.

DETROIT AFRICAN AMERICANS: 1910 - 1939 PERIOD

Social Conditions

The thousands of African Americans who migrated to Detroit from 1910 to 1920 increased the city's African American population by more than 600 percent. Table 3.1 shows the percent increase in the African American population as compared with the percent of Anglo American increase for several North central cities.

Table 3.1: Percent of Black and White Increases

	Negroes 1910	1920	Percent of Negro Increases 1910-20	Percent Of White Increases 1910-20
Cincinnati	19,639	29,636	50.9	8.0
Dayton,OH	4,842	9,029	86.5	28.0
Toledo,OH	1,877	5,690	203.1	42.5
Fort Wayne	572	1,476	158.0	34.3
Canton,OH	291	1,349	363.6	71.7
Gary,IN	383	5,299	1,283.6	205.1
Detroit,MI	5,741	41,532	623.4	106.9
Chicago	44,103	109,594	148.5	21.0

(Turner and Moses 1924)

This large influx primarily of Southern African Americans made Detroit's African American population the fifteenth largest in the United States by 1920 (Deskins 1972:106).

The migration was at its height in May, June, and July, 1917, when 1,000 African Americans a month were arriving in the city. Washington (1920) noted that one day during the summer of 1917, the largest number of African Americans that ever came to Detroit on one train arrived from Birmingham, Alabama. There were over 500 Afrian Americans on this train. Most of the groups arriving were about evenly divided between rural and urban African Americans.

The automotive industry, particularly the Ford company, was the largest employer of African American migrants in

Detroit. Although jobs were relatively easy to obtain, African Americans were frequently given the most menial assignments at the lowest pay with little opportunity to upgrade themselves.

Between 1919 and 1922, African American unemployment in Detroit increased because of the return of veterans looking for work. Detroit's Urban League began to send releases to Southern newspapers urging African Americans not to come to Detroit. Miles (1978) indicated that those African Americans who lacked skills were the first to lose their jobs. Thus in the late 1920s, it became increasingly difficult for unskilled African American workers to find jobs in Detroit.

African Americans who were able to retain their jobs in heavy industries gradually proved their ability to perform on the job and some were able to move from menial laborer positions to semi-skilled and skilled positions. In fact, between April 1922 and April 1923, there was a 70.7% increase in the number of African Americans in skilled positions in Michigan. During the same period, a 62.5% increase occurred in the number of Michigan semi-skilled African Americans. Most of these positions were located in Detroit industries (Miles 1978).

Whether as skilled or unskilled laborers, African Americans were in Detroit to stay. African Americans had proven that they could make the transition from agricultural to industrial work, and were a necessary ingredient in the labor force of the Detroit factories (Miles 1978:106).

Among the 15,000 African Americans employed in the city (57% males and 43% females), ninety-eight percent of

African American women worked primarily in some form of personal service. The remaining 2% were employed as public school teachers. Since most African females were forced to seek employment in the field of personal service, the most desirable and best paid type of personal service jobs were dress-making, hair-dressing or manicuring in the homes of private families. Yet Washington (1920) emphasized that the larger portion of the "cultured" and practically all of the "un-cultured" African American females were employed in the more dull tasks of personal service; namely washing, ironing, housekeeping, and waiting on tables.

Once settled, African Americans wrote their relatives and encouraged them to come to Detroit. According to Washington's study (1920), the size of the average African American family in Detroit, considering only the parents and children was 3.66. Nevertheless, African American households also included extended family members and lodgers. The average African American family therefore con-sisted of 8.83 persons (Washington 1920:117). This relatively large figure is not surprising in the light of the restricted housing available for Detroit African Americans and the cul-tural pattern of African Americans to take on fictive kin or other non-kin sisters and brothers.

The Urban League and several African American churches took the initiative to relieve the housing problem for many African American families (Miles 1978:139). Between 1920 and 1926, African American groups acquired land from the city by subdivision. Subdivision enabled African Americans to purchase lots at a very low price which otherwise could not have been obtained. Fifty-four percent of all lots on record were plotted. Yet as Detroit African Americans gradually expanded their neighborhood and tried to relieve the overcrowding, they met with resistance from some Anglo American residents.

In 1927, an African American doctor, a graduate of Harvard, bought a house in a mostly Anglo American neighborhood. At first he and his wife were harassed and the improvement association planned a strategy to rid the neighborhood of the newcomers. Eventually, the anger subsided and the physician lived in his home without any further incidents (Miles 1978:146). Other African Americans were not as fortunate.

From 1926 to 1939, African Americans made new inroads into the political, economic and social arenas of Detroit. Even the federal government entered the picture and constructed the 941-unit Brewster Home project for low income families in 1937. This project was bounded on the east by Hastings Street, on the west by Beaubien St, and extended for several blocks north and south in the vicinity of Brewster and Mack streets (Boykin 1943:54).

Health Conditions

Since most of Detroit's 120,000 African American residents were congested into one percent of the city's housing, it is not surprising that African Americans were more susceptible to disease than mainstream residents. The deplorable and unsanitary conditions of the lower east side, referred to sarcastically as Paradise Valley, provided an excellent environment for diseases to continue and propagate. The statistics on the general health conditions among Detroit African Americans illustrate this connection.

From 1900 to 1919, for example, the similarities in the death rates for Detroit African Americans and Anglo Americans were apparent. Table 3.2 and 3.3 shows that the most prevalent causes of death among African Americans included pneumonia, tuberculosis of the lungs, heart disease, and syphillis; for Anglo Americans pneumonia, heart disease, and diseases of early childhood and cancer were frequent causes of death. Additionally, African Americans also exhibited a relatively high infant mortality rate (54.7 deaths per 1,000 births).

Table 3.2: Causes of Deaths among Blacks

Causes	Numbers of Deaths	Rate per 100,000
Pneumonia	127	363.0
Tbc of Lungs	67	191.0
Heart Diseases	58	166.0
Disease of Infancy	29	83.0
Diarrhea & Enteritis	22	63.0
Syphillis	20	57.0
Influenza	18	45.0
Cancer	16	46.0
Apoplexy & Cer Hem.	14	43.0

Bright's		
Disease	9	26.0
Typhoid	4	11.0

Table 3.3: Causes of Deaths among Whites

Causes	Numbers of Deaths	Rate per 100,000
Pneumonia	1468	164.0
Heart Diseases	1017	114.0
Diseases of Infancy	971	109.0
Violence	780	87.5
Influenza	774	87.0
Tbc of Lungs	668	77.0
Diarrhea & Enteritis	607	68.0
Cancer	553	62.0
Bright's Disease	421	47.0
Apoplexy & Cer Hem.	385	43.0

(Washington 1920:50)

The major causes of death among African Americans and Anglo Americans can be directly attributed to sociocultural factors. In the most thorough health study conducted upon Detroit African Americans during the 1920s, Washington found that such sociocultural factors as poor housing, lack of health facilities, faulty perceptions of the health care system, shift to a colder environment, and ethnomedical treatment regimens contributed to the high prevalence of diseases.

Since a majority of Detroit's African American population still lived in the Old East Side Negro District, housing was naturally a major predisposing factor for illness. This district contained primarily one and two family framed houses in which an average of nine individuals resided. The large number of occupants in each household, coupled with the unsavory, unsanitary, ill-vented homes along with a poor sewage system would tend to make any population suffer from a high sickness and death rate (Washington 1920).

Related to the diseases which flourished in the unhealthy living quarters was the clothing pattern which was used to adapt to the colder climates. Washington (1920) mentioned that Southern African American migrants often exhibited the habit of wearing too many layers of heavy cotton clothing and wore the same clothes for several months once the cold weather arrived. Women and young children were more likely to dress in this manner because they were often home and not exposed to the so-called "proper clothing pattern" of native Northerns as were the men. From an ecological perspective, it appears that African American women and young children became more susceptible than men for contracting pulmonary diseases primarily because of the following elements: (1) clothing pattern, (2) poorly ventilated homes, (3) unsanitary and poor sewage system, (4) conducive environment for bacillus to flourish, (5) temperature changes, and (6) inadequate diet.

Another living pattern that enabled diseases to develop involved the use of featherbeds and the manner of heating sleeping rooms. Washington (1920) noted that the featherbeds brought in large numbers from the South were perfect incubators for germs since people rarely aired them. Moreover, the custom of heating sleeping rooms with oil stoves and oil lamps throughout the night when they were "over-occupied" and "unventilated" provided an unfavorable influence on the health of the African American migrant.

Another sociocultural and environmental factor which contributed to the high prevalence of diseases among Detroit African Americans was the lack of proper health facilities. Realizing the health problems among African Americans in the United States in 1910, Booker T. Washington established National Negro Health Week. The "Health Week" was actively promoted in the Detroit African American community during the 1920s with health lectures and special programs. Yet, availability and access to proper health facilities were often denied to many Detroit African Americans. The fact that during this period several hospitals refused to admit African American patients, and only one Anglo American controlled hospital allowed African American physicians to practice in their facility, compounded the Detroit African American health problem (Turner and Moses 1924 and Miles 1978:205).

Disturbed about the lack of adequate health care available to the thousands of African Americans in Detroit, a number of

African American physicians and laymen formed the Dunbar Memorial Hospital Association in 1918 (Miles 1978). The specific purpose of the association was to study sanitation and related issues, and to maintain a hospital and a school of nursing. Dunbar Hospital was especially important because it was mainly concerned with the health of the African American community and provided an opportunity for African American physicians to practice medicine. Mercy Hospital, founded in 1916, was the only other hospital serving the African American community. This small private hospital, about half the size of Dunbar, was never able to make a significant contribution to the community because it had only 25 beds and a very small staff.

Apart from the Detroit Board of Health's special clinic for African American infants, Detroit African Americans had only the use of the outpatient clinics in most of the city's hospitals. Although African American patients preferred to be treated by African American physicians, Detroit African Americans still opted for outpatient services or used traditional folk healers. Ironically, the most prevalent diseases in the African American community required hospitalization for effective treatment. Miles (1978) and Turner et al. (1924) emphasized that because of the inaccessibility to local health facilities and the inability to receive effective treatment, many Detroit African Americans as well as the remaining general public died from pneumonia and tuberculosis.

A common occurrence in all groups, namely the fear of hospitals, caused many African Americans to avoid using mainstream health care facilities (Washington 1920). This fear was based upon African American's perceptions that the hospital's physicians practiced experimental laboratory tests on patients. Thus, cultural beliefs based upon fact or misperceptions concerning the health care system were another sociocultural factor which affected Detroit African American's utilization pattern of public hospitals.

Not surprisingly, the use of traditional folk healers (alternative health practitioners) and remedies became an integral part of the health care strategy among Detroit African Americans. Washington (1920) stated that a large proportion of African Americans who were ill depended entirely upon folk healers for treatment. He identified a number of "herb doctors" who operated in several African American sections of the city.

Spiritualists, referred to as "Divine Healers," were also prospering in the community with their ethnomedical therapy of "laying-on-of-hands." Washington (1920) documented the following:

"One of these healers started in business only a few months ago charging 50 cents a treatment. He has built up such a following that he is now charging from $2.00 to $25.00, according to the amount he thinks a patient will be able to pay. His office is always full of sick Negroes who get up early in the morning to be first in line when his place of business opens." (Washington 1920)

A number of Anglo Americans was also observed attending the facilities of the Divine Healers.

Because of the inaccessibility to mainstream health care facilities and the complete reliance upon alternative health practitioners, a number of serious diseases was simply undetected. Unfortunately, many of these diseases brought death to the victim before proper medical attention could intervene.

Although a number of sociocultural factors were acting against the health of African American Detroiters, there were some significant improvements. For example, once African Americans received a higher salary, they provided more adequately for their family's physical needs; thereby reducing the death rates associated with infectious diseases. The increase in the number of African American physicians (5 in 1910 to 27 in 1925) directly contributed by the Board of Health which incorporated African American social workers and nurses to advise and educate the community on proper clothing and diet supplied a new medium to combat serious diseases (Turner and Moses 1924). During this period, Detroit African Americans needed a massive health education program to acquaint them with available health facilities and healthy living patterns.

This health care problem did not confine itself to Detroit. It also held true not only for Detroit African Americans but other ethnic groups throughout the United States (Elzy 1927:175). The following summarizes the attitude among many African American migrants in 1927.

"While things look dark now in Northern communities, where there are a great many Negroes who recently came

from the South, their coming here will mean much to the future development of the entire race. They are being exposed to sanitary conditions which are entirely new to them. They are coming in contact with people who have higher standards of living than their own, hence they will naturally absorb at least some of their ideas. They are more and more seeking the proper medical advice and here they also get hygenic information. They seem eager to learn, and are very teachable. If they had remained in the rural South they would have been subjected to its lack of opportunity indefinitely. In about a decade from now, the Negroes who came North this year will have a remarkable positive change, and this is encouraging."
(McGhee 1927:178)

In sum, the 1910 - 1939 period reflected a era of prosperity and disappointment for the new African American migrants. The opportunities of employment in the Northern urban cities had its negative effects on the health status of Detroit African Americans. Nevertheless, Southern African Americans continued to arrive in Detroit by the thousands.

DETROIT AFRICAN AMERICANS: 1940 - 1964 PERIOD

Social Conditions
Because of the effects of WWI and the increased mechanization of Southern agricultural system, African Americans migrated to Northern industrial cities in huge numbers. Between 1940 to 1966, 3.7 million African Americans left the South (Palmer 1967). Within a ten year period (1940 - 1950)

the African American population in Detroit doubled from 149,119 to 300,506 (Detroit Urban League 1965:3). Only Baltimore, Washington D.C., Chicago, and New Orleans experienced higher percentage increases of African Americans in their city's population.

The doubling of Detroit's African American population resulted in the "White exodus" to the suburbs and limited spacial expansion of the community. Although African Americans acquired more housing within the city and the suburbs, the condition of this housing was substantially inferior to Anglo American residents (Detroit Urban League 1965). Figure 3.1 shows the available African American housing projects in Detroit.

For example, over three-quarters of the African Americans occupied housing was over thirty years old as opposed to one-half of Anglo American occupied units. In the suburbs, only one-fifth of the Anglo American population lived in housing more than thirty years old; and this housing was largely unavailable to African Americans. Despite the ability of some African Americans to move into the apartments, flats, and houses of Anglo Americans, a major portion of the blighted housing was occupied still by African Americans (Detroit Urban League 1965).

During the ensuing years, the housing situation changed significantly. Between 1950 and 1960, no fewer than eighty-three additional census tracts became available to African Americans compared to twenty-four in the previous decade. The most notable extension of the African American community happened in the northwest section of Detroit. Figure

Figure 3.1   Black Housing Projects in Detroit

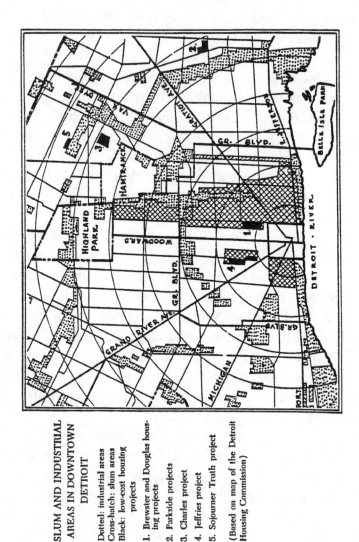

(Lee 1943:24)

SLUM AND INDUSTRIAL
AREAS IN DOWNTOWN
DETROIT

Dotted: industrial areas
Cross-hatch: slum areas
Black: low-cost housing
   projects

1. Brewster and Douglas housing projects
2. Parkside projects
3. Charles project
4. Jeffries project
5. Sojourner Truth project

(Based on map of the Detroit
Housing Commission)

3.2 depicts the non-White distribution and subcommunities in the Detroit Metropolitan area (see appendix).

As the African American population expanded, the residences of Detroit African American middle class and lower classes separated (Henderson 1965). Middle-class African Americans moved closer to their Anglo American counterparts, whereas lower-class African Americans remained in the original African American settlements. Occupational status and educational level were related directly to this pattern of African American expansion.

Yet as the northwesterly movements of African Americans continued, so did the exodus of Anglo Americans from the city of Detroit. By 1960, the total population of Detroit had declined from 1,849,568 to 1,670,000 of which 70.8% (1,545,847) were Anglo American. From 1950 to 1960, the total population declined by 9.7%, the Anglo American population declined by nearly 23.5%; thereby increasing the African American percentage of Detroit's population to 29 percent. Thousands of Anglo American residents thus left the inner-city for suburban areas (Detroit Urban League 1965:3).

Those who remained in the inner-city were more likely than suburban residents to live in substandard housing, to have completed eight years of school or less, and to be employed as laborers and service workers. According to Kornhauser's (1952) survey of attitudes of Detroit people toward the conditions in the city, respondents indicated that housing (51%) and Black-White relations (46%) were the two biggest problems. Given these factors coupled with the high crime rate and the chronic unemployment among inner-city residents, African American Detroiters finally decided to publicize their plight.

On Sunday June 23, 1964, Rev. Martin Luther King joined African American Detroiters in a march designed to raise the consciousness of city, state, and federal officials concerning the deplorable conditions and mistreatment of human rights which persisted against minorities in Detroit and in other regions of the United States (Miles 1978:242). These pleas for jobs, fair housing, and civil rights were not heeded. The lack of action by city officials led eventually to more traumatic events years later.

Health Conditions

During this period, the health conditions and health status of Detroit African Americans were directly linked to their residence pattern. As one would expect, the highest rates for all forms of diseases occurred in inner-city areas: in those areas with the highest concentration of African American residencies.

The high prevalence of disease, nevertheless, declined as African Americans moved further from the inner-city. This trend suggests how sociodemographics affects health status. As more African Americans migrated to suburban regions, their health status was better than that of those who remained in the inner-city. Thus, an increase in income and education and a healthier physical environment enabled many Detroit African Americans to achieve some economic and political gains and also an improved health status.

DETROIT AFRICAN AMERICANS: 1965 - PRESENT

Social Conditions

By 1967, a comparatively large and relatively prosperous African American middle class had slowly but surely gained acceptance in the economic and political life of the city. A higher percentage of African Americans owned homes in Detroit than in any other large Northern city. Although Anglo American-owned real estate firms and mortgage companies still exercised control over the direction and rate of African American geographical expansion, larger areas of the city became available for African American settlement. Such advances as a growing economic power, liberal Supreme Court decision relating to housing, and a coalition of African American leaders backed by powerful automotive labor unions supplied a political base for the large African American population. However, as one sector of the African American population prospered, others did less well.

The complaints of many Detroit African Americans in the early 1960s concerning unemployment, inadequate housing, high crime rates, police harassment, and a host of other social ills resulted in feelings of hopelessness, fear, and anger (Cunningham 1972:205). These feelings were vented ultimately in the riot of 1967 (July). Sparked by a police raid on a African American "blind pig" (an illegal drinking place), African Americans looted (1,700 stores) and burned (419) a large number of establishments. Federal troops were required to squelch the uprising and a riot control program was implemented in the city.

The city's action prompted the following statement from John Diamond (Chairman of the Detroit Mayor's Committee for Human Resources Development):

"The focus on riot control and prevention emphasizes and promotes hysteria, fear, and the psychology that pre-conditions our citizenry for further civic dis- turbance. We will repeat the areas needing support and emphasis knowing that you are already aware of them; namely, job opportunities for all, adequate low cost housing and quality education for the inner-city. Unless there is greater and greater emphasis and promotion of the programs that are fundamental to the community needs the results are disastrous. The adequate reallocation of community resources toward jobs, housing, and education must be your message to the community if we are to see the improvements we all desire."
(Diamond 1967:1)

By the early 1970s, additional housing became available for Detroit African Americans. Educational opportunities, training programs, and accessibility to health care facilities also increased.

From 1970 to the present, the city of Detroit has continued its racial transition. Between 1970 and 1980, the percentage of African Americans increased by 22 percent (44% - 66%). Currently, Detroit's racial composition is approximately 67 percent African American and 33 percent Anglo American. Not only did the percentage of African Americans increase within the city, but those who were economically and medically dependent also increased (20.1% - 29.7%) (Comprehensive Health Planning Council 1981).

Health Conditions
Related to these socioeconomic trends are the five leading causes of death at present in Detroit: (1) heart disease, (2) malignant neoplasms, (3) cerebrovascular disease, (4) homicide, and (5) accidents (Greater Detroit Area Health Council 1983). The first three causes of death at present in Detroit mirror the major causes of death in urban and urbanized societies worldwide (Kaplan 1988). Additionally, Detroit's infant mortality rate (22 per 1,000 births) is one of the highest in the nation. The health and economic problems which presently afflict Detroit African Americans and other ethnic groups are a direct consequence of decades of political, economic, and social neglect by those who legislate public programs.

CONCLUSION

This cultural-historical review shows how the region's economic, social, and political climate affected Detroit African Americans' health status and their use of mainstream health care facilities. Cultural and ethnic groups migrating to urban areas must decide whether: to adhere to their own values and behavior patterns; to integrate certain values and norms of the urban population with theirs; or to adapt to the values, norms, customs, and behaviors of the population among whom they have moved.

When African American families migrated from the South during the 1800s and 1900s, they did so primarily because of the persistent decline of the Southern rural economy and the rigid discrimination in employment, housing, education, and health care. Upon arrival in the Northern cities, these migrants were able to achieve a certain degree of economic, social, and political success. Yet, as with all immigrant groups in a new setting, the reality was different from the expectation. Urbanization resulted in greater differentiation in the economic and social stratification of the African American population with corresponding variations in family structure, educational achievement, and health care patterns.

Chapter 4

RESEARCH METHODS

INTRODUCTION

Inductive reasoning proceeds by a continous chain of questions and anwers, beginning at the base of a pyamid with data from direct observations and ending with an abstract proposition (Wagenaar 1981:50). While volunteering at a large urban hospital in Detroit, I observed numerous client-staff encounters. As the months passed, it became apparent that the client and the health staff had two different "understandings" regarding the etiology of an illness.

From the client's perspective, uncertainty about the course of his/her problem is part of the illness; whereas among health personnel, the organ pathology (disease) is often most important. In client-staff encounters, health staff primarily ask symptom-oriented questions related to perceived diseases; whereas the client expresses disease as a perception and experience of everyday activities.

After 4 months of direct observations, I investigated the concept of "illness behavior." This behavior is part of the health care seeking process which involves the way a person evaluates and acts in response to perceived symptoms of a disease (Kirscht 1974:387). Once the basis of this behavior was understood, the implementation of a two-phased study utilizing the United Health Organization's facilities for interviewing available during the operation of the 1985 and 1986 health screenings was undertaken.

ETHNOGRAPHIC RESEARCH

Ethnographic research has a long and continuing history in cultural anthropology to investigate human behavior. To understand and describe a cultural and/or ethnic group, anthropologist engage in ethnographic fieldwork. Fieldwork refers to firsthand observation of human societies - as a means of gathering data and testing hypotheses generated by theories. This means living with people, eating their food, learning their language, listening to gossip, examining the items they produce, asking questions, recording answers, and above all simply watching the people's daily routines and interactions. The second phase of this study used ethnographic methods such as: (1) informal and semi-structured interviews, (2) individual health profiles, and (3) traditional fieldwork techniques.

Informal and Semi-Structured Interviews

The informal interview (open-ended) was a part of the ethnographic method. This casual question-and-answer session encourages informant to follow his/her own train of thought, wherever it might lead; thereby providing information about the subject from his/her viewpoint and experiences. This interview technique was particularly important because it enabled the informant's ideas, world views, and information be revealed rather than those of the interviewer.

The semi-structured interview, by contrast, is a combination of both an informal (open) and a structured type of interview. It is designed to elicit both definitive and unexpected kinds of information from the interviewee. Such examples of semi-structured questions were: (1) Some people have not sought physician care when they should have; Are you one of these persons and why?; and (2) Once you became aware that your blood pressure was high, what did you do about it and why? Although the questions were predetermined by the researcher, the respondent has the ability to elaborate on certain issues.

Individual Health Profiles
The individual health profile method was chosen as another method for this study as a special way of obtaining a chronological sequence (short or long) of an individual's ideas and experiences from their particular viewpoint. The 27 individual health profiles yielded insightful information that was not obtainable by the semi-structured interviews.

In this study, the purposes of individual health profiles were to: (1) obtain intimate and detailed knowledge about the individual; (2) identify health care and illness patterns; (3) identify actual and potential factors leading to illness; and (4) gain a comprehensive view of the individual's environment and lifestyle over short or long periods of time; and (5) generalize from the individual to the population. All of these qualitative research methods were used to serve as additional avenues toward understanding the health patterns among the sample of Detroit African Americans.

THE 1985 HEALTH SCREENING SURVEY: FIRST PHASE

Procedure

The first phase of this study was designed to determine the individual's ethnomedical beliefs regarding hypertension, their reasons for using or avoiding available health services, and the factors health professionals can use in modifying a client's health care practices. In cooperation with United Health Organization's Project Health-O-Rama, clients of the health screenings at seven sites in the Detroit Metropolitan area were interviewed. These sites included community health centers, churches, and malls.

In the data collection technique, both structured and semi-structured interviews are used. Usually I interviewed volunteering informants after nurses screened them for high blood pressure. Most interviews lasted approximately 10-15 minutes; although others took considerably longer because of the open-ended format of semi-structured interviews. I also took the role of a blood pressure screener when there were too few health care professionals at the screening site.

Semi-Structured Questionnaires

Instruments used in this study were Becker's Health Belief Questionnaire (1977) and Spielberger's State Anxiety Inventory (1970) with slight modifications made by the researcher. Both instruments were modified chiefly because of limited interviewing time and appropriateness of the questions with each client.

The Health Belief questions sought to determine: (1) perceived seriousness and susceptibility of hypertension, (2) perceived health benefits and barriers to screening programs, and (3) the source of perceived internal or external cues to action. Other questions addressed sociodemographic characteristics and adherence to mainstream preventive health care regimens (see appendix). Figure 4.1 depicts the factors associated with the Health Belief model (see appendix). The Health Belief section totaled 19 questions.

Spielberger's State Anxiety Inventory (A - state) and the Health Belief questionnaire were used to determine the possible relationship of psychosocial and sociocultural factors with the informant's blood pressure level and health care seeking pattern. Speilberger, in his State-Trait Anxiety Inventory (STAI), calculates anxiety by: (1) observing the patient and developing sentences which described the behavior associated with varying degrees of anxiety; (2) interviewing the subject and obtaining statements from them their level of anxiety; and (3) having the subjects rate their own anxiety.

The researcher used Spielberger's STAI questionnaire in this study for three main reasons: namely (1) to examine more underlying components of anxiety than other anxiety (stress) questionnaires; (2) to provide an appropriate method to inquire about individual social stressors; and (3) to fit the limited time restrictions with each informant (Newmark 1972; Bauer et al. 1983; Byrne and Whyte 1983; Johnson et al. 1983; and Adams et al. 1986).

The STAI A-state scale consisted of twenty statements (e.g., "I am jittery;""I feel rested"). Informants are asked to describe how they feel at a particular moment by rating themselves on the following four-point scale: (1) Not at all; (2) Somewhat; (3) Moderately so; and (4) Very much so.

The STAI A-state scoring system was designed so that if an informant answered "Very much so," the statement was scored a 4. The values of A-state ranged from 1 to 4 with a maximum total of 80. In some items, scoring in the opposite direction was required. For example, feeling "Not at all" - calm was scored a 4 while feeling "Not at all" - tense scored a 1 (Spielberger 1970). Spielberger's (1970) guidelines for mean A-state score in stress condition (40.87) is significantly higher than in the nonstress condition (38.98).

The Sample

The sample consisted of 183 informants, eighty-two were African Americans. There were 119 females and 64 males ranging in age from 19 to 85 years. This sample reflected primarily the type of clientele attending Project Health-O-Rama health screenings (mostly older adults) and those who tended to volunteer for research projects. Most interviews were conducted after nurses screened clients for high blood pressure.

Data from the interviews were coded and entered onto the computer at Wayne State University (Detroit, Michigan) using the Statistical Package for Social Sciences (SPSSX) (SPSSX Guide 1983). The focus of data analyses sought to determine the factors related to blood pressure level and health care seeking behavior. The data were analyzed by using standard parametric statistics such as t-test, Pearson correlations, and multiple regressions to test the health belief indices, anxiety scores, and demographic variables.

THE 1986 HEALTH SCREENING: SECOND PHASE

Procedure

The initial research at the 1986 health screenings paralled the methods used in 1985. Additionally, in the 1986 study more time was allocated in the collection of individual health profiles. These strategies sought to obtain in-depth and personal accounts of an individual's illness and behavior. Data in the second phase of the study was collected over twelve months, and included informant-oriented and observation-oriented methods. The sequence was as follows:

1. the first seven months: consisted of informal interviews and unstructured observations;

2. the next four weeks: included semi-structured interviews and

3. the final four months: included informal interviews and individual health profiles.

In cooperation with the United Health Organization, I collected ethnographic data from African Americans residing in and around the nine randomly selected health screening sites in the Detroit Metropolitan area. These sites were also community health centers, churches, and malls. From September 1985 through March 1986, I collected data informally from informants via the snowball sampling (i.e..networking) method (Bailey 1982). This method consists of interviewing persons in the designated communities, who in turn recommended other persons who could be interviewed and so on. I was aware that this technique might not obtain a true representation of the population. However, the general and key informants were primarily local community leaders, health professionals, and residents. Although an individual frequently serves in both roles (general and key informant), an important difference exists between the two.

General informants provide the researcher with personal accounts of what they thought, they saw, and did during some event or about some issue. In contrast, key informants provide descriptions of the group or research setting as a whole (Fitzpatrick 1981). Thus, general informants discuss personal experiences, while key informants provide insightful cultural data.

During the April 1986 health screenings (4 weeks), data were gathered using semi-structured interviews. As was done in the 1985 health screenings (1st phase), I interviewed general informants who volunteered after nurses screened them for high blood pressure. These individuals (258) were asked a series of questions about their beliefs, values, and behaviors regarding high blood pressure. In addition, demographic and sociocultural data was obtained as were responses to the Health Belief Questionnaire and Spielberger's State Anxiety Questionnaire. General and key informants included clients and health professionals of the local health screening and non-clients in the immediate vicinity of the local health screening.

These procedures continued from May to August 1986 at three of the nine sampled health screening sites. Individuals providing health profiles were non-clients and clients of local health screenings and site chairmen/coordinators of the sampled health screening sites.

The Sample
The sample consisted of 203 African Americans of which 176 were semi-structured interviews (68 - 39% were male and 108 - 61% female) and 27 individual health profiles and 82 Anglo Americans (semi-structured interviews). The semi-structured interviews and individual health profiles were analyzed by focusing on different cognitive and identifiable themes and patterns of living or of behavior to determine whether certain behavioral patterns could be discerned. The patterns (small units of behavior) and themes (large unit of analysis) derived from the qualitative data helped to obtain a full picture of the individual within contrasting lifestyles (Leininger 1985).

Guidelines for Informal Interviews and Health Profiles
The informal interviews and health profiles followed various formats depending upon the circumstances surrounding each encounter with a informant. I used a general guideline for each interview. The 27 individual health profiles followed this format:

1. Tell me a little bit about yourself.

2. Let us talk about where you were born and what you remember about your early days of growing up, keeping well, or experiencing illnesses.

3. I would like to hear your general philosophy of keeping well and how you believe your religion, political, and cultural values have helped (or hindered) your life goals and health. Can you tell me what beliefs or values have especially guided you to remaining well or becoming ill? (Give examples)

4. Throughout your life, what factors seemed to keep you going, living, or establishing healthy patterns of living for yourself and others.

5. Was there any ocassion in which mainstream society affected your utilization of health care services?

6. What would you suggest to the site coordinators of U.H.O. to increase the African American communities participation of the local health screenings?

The sample of 27 individual health profiles (19 women and 8 men) was selected by networking with key informants: some informants had participated in the semi-structured interviews during the health screening; whereas others were recruited from local churches and senior citizens outreach facilities. Data collection of health profiles also varied in time and place. For instance, most health profile interviews were conducted and completed at the health screening site within a two hour period. Others, however, were conducted at the informants' home and lasted two to three hours each day for approximately five days.

When an informant had a particular health problem (essential hypertension), I elicited the individual's explanations with questions such as the following:

1. What do you call your problem? What name does it have?

2. What do you think has caused your problem?

3. Why do you think it started when it did?

4. What does your sickness do to you? How does it work?

5. How severe is it? Will it have a short or a long course?

6. What do you fear most about your sickness?

7. What are the chief problems your sickness has caused for you?

8. What kinds of treatment do you think you should receive? What are the most important results you hope to receive from the treatment?

9. Who do you ask to help when you are sick?

10. Where do you go for help first?

11. If that does not work, where do you go?

12. What does being "healthy" mean to you?

13. What do you do to maintain good health?

Those who considered themselves "healthy" were only asked to elaborate upon questions 12 and 13.

Informal interviews were also conducted among site coordinators and site chairmen of United Health Organization to examine their opinions about the success or failure of the 1986 health screenings. Twenty-two semi-structured questions addressed issues such as:

1. Did the screening accomplish its goal?

2. Why do you think some sites were less successful than others?

3. Do you think it's necessary to implement any special intervention strategies for the young or for different ethnic groups?

4. How would you effectively mobilize a "hard" to reach group?

5. Why do you think some people are more mainstream preventative-oriented than others?

6. What are the future goals or direction for Project Health-O-Rama?

Data from the analysis of the informal interviews and the individual health profiles of the local community residents and site coordinators/chairmen was later integrated with the quantitative data (structured interviews) from the health screenings to produce a holistic view of the factors which influenced health care seeking and also provided data on essential intervention strategies which should be implemented in the African American community.

In sum, the ethnographic method was the principal research method used during the 1986 health screening. Additionally, the individual health profiles provided a cultural relativistic perspective of the informant's beliefs and health care patterns with regard to high blood pressure and the adaptive strategies African Americans use to maintain health despite varying socioeconomic constraints.

Chapter 5

HEALTH EXPRESSIONS: A QUANTITATIVE ANALYSIS

INTRODUCTION

To understand the health care utilization patterns of Detroit African Americans, I analyzed the data obtained from informants following each phase of the study. Data analyses are presented for the 1985 and 1986 health screenings. Quantitative and qualitative data analyses provided the basis of this study's findings. These findings established an identifiable pattern of health care seeking among Detroit African Americans regarding their ethnomedical beliefs of hypertension.

THE 1985 HEALTH SCREENING

Characteristic of Sample

The sample of informants who participated in the semi-structured interviews consisted of 69 men (39%) and 119 women (61%) ranging in ages from 18 to 90 years. The range of income was between $10,000 to $14,999 per year (Table 5.1). The identified ethnic groups were as follows: 4 Italian Americans, 20 German Americans, 16 Irish Americans, 2 Phillipinos, 8 Appalachians, 82 African Americans, 1 Hispanic American, 1 Asian American, 1 Native American, and 48 Anglo Americans. Because of the small number of ethnic groups, such groups as Italian Americans, German

Americans, Irish Americans and Appalachians with Anglo
Americans and Hispanic Americans, Asian Americans, Na-
tive Americans and Phillipinos have here been combined as
Others to provide a statistical comparison between Anglo
Americans and African Americans.

TABLE 5.1:   **1985 Demographic Distribution**

	N	White(%)	N	Black(%)
Sex of Informant				
Male	35	(41%)	29	(34%)
Female	61	(59%)	53	(66%)
	96		82	
Informant's Age (Mean)		61.2		56.7
Total Family Income (Mode Ranges)		$10,000-14,999		$5,000-9,999

*An Addition 5 informants were classified
as others.

The sample consisted of 68 hypertensives (25 African
Americans, 40 Anglo Americans, and 3 Others) and 115 normotensives (57 African Americans, 56 Anglo Americans, and
2 Others). Systolic blood pressures ranged from 161 mmHg
to 110 mmHg and diastolic blood pressures ranged from 92

mmHg to 68 mmHg. Distribution between male and female blood pressures were 133/80 mmHg and 128/78 mmHg respectively. Of the two generalized ethnic groups, Anglo Americans' blood pressure was 129/78 mmHg and African Americans' blood pressure was 126/76 mmHg. There were no significant differences between any of the groups.

Health Beliefs and Hypertension

One of the major objectives of this study was to analyze the informants' ethnomedical beliefs regarding hypertension. A series of questions examined the participants' and non-participants' beliefs about the following major attributes of high blood pressure: (1) its causes; (2) its signs or symptoms, and (3) its treatment.

Informants were asked what word or words would you use for a person who has a raised blood pressure level? A majority of the sample (52.2%) referred to the problem of having a raised blood pressure level as "high blood pressure." Those who answered "other" used the folk term "high blood." Thus, most individuals identified with the allopathic terminology of hypertension.

Ninety-one percent of the informants believed that high blood pressure was caused by emotional worry. The other most frequently stated causes of hypertension were obesity, high salt diet, cholesterol (fatty foods), and heredity. Old age and lack of exercise were not considered major factors contributing to high blood pressure.

If emotional worry was perceived as the major cause of their heightened blood pressure, informants believed that once the psychosocial stress was alleviated, their blood pressure would return to normal. Some informants, therefore, disregarded their anti-hypertensive medication since they preferred an ethno-care approach ('folk' or 'emic' caring practices) in diagnosing their major stressors. This health care action was also a symbolic response (maintain ethnic health care practices) to avoid the dependency to mainstream anti-hypertensive medication.

Contrary to physicians' and nurses' assertions (American Heart Association), fifty-percent of the informants felt that they could tell when their blood pressure was high or slightly elevated. Significantly more of the sample associated symptoms with high blood pressure such as headaches, dizziness, warmth, seeing spots, and tension (Chi square=41.9, df=24, p=.01). Informants who experienced symptoms used these signs as "markers" or "signals" to begin or temporarily increase the dosage of their anti-hypertensive medication (Chi square=15.9, df=8, p=.01).

Although significant differences between ethnic groups' perception of symptoms in this 1985 sample were not apparent, other demographic data exhibited meaningful variance (variability). Women, for instance, stated that they could tell when their blood pressure was high (67%) more often than men (55%) (Chi square=3.3, df=1, p=.05). Informants in the 35 to 55 yr.-age group were aware of more symptoms that those in the 18 to 34 or 56 to 90 yr.-age groups (one-way analysis, p=.05). In addition, a comparison between hypertensive and normotensive informants indicated that significantly more hypertensives (75%) claimed to be able to feel when their blood pressure became elevated than normotensives (25%, Chi square=13.9, df=1, p=.0003). Thus as expected, once an individual is labeled "hypertensive," he/she pays more attention to the perceived symptoms associated with high blood pressure.

The most startling of informants' beliefs about hypertension emerged from a consideration of the treatment therapy. Although most informants realized the perceived health benefits of controlling one's blood pressure (89%, less likely to have a stroke and 90% less likely to have a heart attack), use of mainstream anti-hypertensive medication was not considered necessary.

Of those whose income range was less than $5,000 a year, fifty percent stated that anti-hypertensive medication was inexpensive primarily because people in this age group received their medication free or as part of medicaid at very reduced prices. Between ethnic groups, however, significantly more African Americans (47%) than Anglo Americans (31%) commented that blood pressure medication was indeed expensive (Chi square=2.55, df=1, p=.01).

Demographics and Blood Pressure
An hierarchial stepwise regression determined the following factors contributing to the variance in the informants' blood pressure: (1) age, (2) income level, and (3) ethnicity (Table 5.2). Age accounted for approximately 14 percent (B=.48, p=.008) and income level nearly 28 percent (B=-.38, p=.03) of the variance in systolic blood pressure. Although ethnic

identity was not significant, it did contribute to a portion of the variance (9%, B=.30). This statistical analyses suggest that those who were older with low incomes (inverse relationship) tended to exhibit higher blood pressure levels. A multiple regression for diastolic blood pressure showed no significant variability.

Informants who indicated that they had been previously diagnosed as hypertensive showed significantly higher systolic (t=5.56, df=178, p=.0001) and diastolic (t=3.96, df=178, p=.0001) blood pressures than normotensives.

Table 5.2: Multiple Regression for Systolic BP

Independent Variables	Beta	t	p=
Occupation	.12	.70	.48
Unemployed	-.06	-.35	.72
Income	-.38	-2.24	.03*
Education	-.18	1.52	.13
Age	.48	2.83	.008*
Sex	-.02	-.15	.87
Ethnicity	.30	1.52	.13

Multiple R = .52
R square = .27
Adjusted R = .22   Standard Error = 16.0
  square

Psychosocial Stress: State Anxiety

Spielberger's State Anxiety Inventory served to determine the effects of perceived stress with the informant's health care seeking behavior. As discussed in Chapter 4, this instrument was used for two main reasons: (1) it examined more under-lying components of anxiety (stress) than other question-naires and (2) it provided an appropriate method to inquire about individual social stressors.

A one-way analysis of variance determined whether dif-ferences occurred between groups. Mean state anxiety for the population was 37.6 (SD=7.0). State anxiety scores for males was significantly higher 39.14 (SD=7.7) than that for females 36.4 (SD=6.2, t=2.3, df=182, p=.04). Mean state anxiety for African Americans (38.7, SD=7.0) was not significantly higher than Anglo Americans' mean scores (36.7, SD=6.6).

Although there was no significant correlation between blood pressure level and state anxiety scores, the relationship was in the direction expected (p=.15). Some notable differences, nonetheless, occurred between groups. Male state anxiety was significantly higher than was that for females. Second, differences in mean state anxiety between the 18 to 35 year-age group and 36 to 55 year-age group was significant (t=2.4, df=182, p=.01). The mean state anxiety score was 39.7 (SD=7.9) for the younger age group and 36.1 (SD=6.3) for the middle age group. The 56 to 90 yr.-age group had a mean state score closer to the 36 to 55 yr.-age group (36.7, SD=6.3). Thus, younger individuals experienced higher anxiety levels than did older ones.

The combined effects of being unemployed with a low in-come are reflected in mean state anxiety scores. State anxiety scores were negatively correlated with income (r=-.15) and unemployed informants had significantly higher mean state anxiety scores (39.5, SD=7.8) than employed informants

(36.9, SD=6.7). This difference was statistically significant (t=2.03, df=155, p=.04).

Utilization of Health Screening

The majority of the informants (hypertensives and normotensives) in this study (56%) had not previously attended a Project Health-O-Rama health screening. Those who have used this health screening previously were significantly more likely to be employed and were in the 56 to 75+ yr.-age group (64%) (Chi square=25.2, df=2, p=.0001). These characteristics reflected the typical Project Health-O-Rama participant.

A hierarchical stepwise regression conducted on the health belief indices indicated that perceived costs (physical - barriers, psychological - state anxiety, and financial - income level) provided the most variance of all the health belief items. Approximately 10 percent of the variance can be explained by these indices. At this step, of the three perceived cost variables, state anxiety was most significant.

THE 1986 HEALTH SCREENING

Characteristics of Sample

Table 5.3 presents the demographic distributions for the entire sample. Of the 285 general and key informants, 176 African Americans and 82 Anglo Americans completed the semi-structured interviews. The 27 individual health profiles were all conducted among African Americans. Other demographics included 86 (49%) married, 70 (40%) belonging to the 36 to 55 year-age group, mean income ranging from \$10,000 to \$14,999 per year, and mean educational level - high school or equivalent (see appendix, Tables 5.4 - 5.11).

TABLE 5.3: 1986 Demographic Distribution

	N	African American(%)	N	Anglo American(%)
Sex of Informant				
Male	68	(39%)	24	(29%)
Female	108	(61%)	58	(71%)
	176	(100%)	82	(100%)

Total Family Income (Mean Range)
         \$10,000-\$14,999   \$35,000 or more Age
(Mean Range)
         36 - 55 years   56 or older

Educational Level (Mean)
   High School or Equiv.   High School or Equiv.

*Sample Note: An additional 27 individual life histories
   (African Americans:similar sociodemographics)

In addition, a small sample of Anglo-Americans (82) participated in the semi-structured interviews as the control group. Sex distribution was similar to the African American sample. Twenty-four (29%) were male and 58 (71%) female. The Anglo American group, however, differed from the

African American in that more were married and the majority belonged to an older age group (Table 5.3).

Systolic blood pressures ranged from 240 mmHg to 80 mmHg and diastolic blood pressures ranged from 60 mmHg to 130 mmHg. There were no significant differences between ethnic groups (see appendix, Tables 5.12 and 5.13). African Americans, however, were significantly more likely to have been diagnosed as hypertensive (55%) than Whites (41%). Hypertensives had a mean blood pressure of 141/84 mmHg compared to normotensives' (125/77 mmHg).

Blood pressures between males and females showed a significant difference in diastolic blood pressure (t=2.27, df=255, p=.02). Males' mean systolic and diastolic blood pressure was slightly higher (135/82 mmHg) than females (131/79 mmHg). The apparent statistical difference of diastolic blood pressure between males and females was inconclusive after t-test analysis (t=2.27, df=255, p=.02) (see appendix, Tables 5.14 - 5.19).

Health Beliefs and Hypertension

As with the 1985 survey, a series of questions addressed the individual's ethnomedical beliefs regarding hypertension: (1) its causes; (2) its signs or symptoms, and (3) its treatment. Semi-structured interviews were conducted among 176 African Americans and 82 Anglo Americans at various health screening sites.

Specifically, more African Americans (97%) than Anglo Americans (93%) believed that emotional worry (psychosocial stress) caused high blood pressure (Chi square=6.4, df=2, p=.03). Secondly, more Anglo Americans (65%) than African Americans (53%) acknowledged that age contributed to a high blood pressure level (Chi square=5.6, df=2, p=.05). Finally, African Americans (60%) were less likely than Anglo Americans (91%) to believe that hereditary components contributed to an individual's high blood pressure level (Chi square=26.2, df=2, p=.000).

An hierarchical multiple regression assessed which factors contributed the most variance to the individual's belief that symptoms were associated with high blood pressure. Of all these factors (age, sex, ethnicity, total family income, and education), only ethnicity approached significance (B=.11, p=.09). In fact, African American females (67%) were significantly more likely than Anglo American females (51%) to claim to perceive symptoms with a heightened blood pressure level (Chi square=3.8, df=1, p=.04). No significant difference occurred between African American (57%) and Anglo American males (42%, p=.20). In general, African Americans exhibited an ethnomedical belief that individuals can determine whether their "blood" is high or even low.

Another finding concerns the informant's beliefs about mainstream anti-hypertensive treatment. An overwhelming majority of both ethnic groups (95% Anglo Americans and 92% African Americans) recognized the perceived benefits of controlling high blood pressure. Nevertheless, African American males and females were significantly less likely than Anglo males and females to treat their elevated blood pressure with a prescribed anti-hypertension medication. Those who answered the question, "Do you need high blood pressure medication only when you have a headache, feel dizzy, or feel sick, 32% of African American female informants answered "yes" compared to 9% of the Anglo American female informants (Chi square=11.8, df=2, p=.002). The significant difference reflects possibly fear of consequences.

A multiple regression analysis examined the variables contributing the most variance to the perceived costs of anti-hypertensive medication. These 7 variables (age, sex, ethnicity, total family income, occupation, employment status, and education) accounted for 12% of the total variance associated with the perceived high cost of medication. Of these, total family income (B=.15, p=.03), sex (B=.21, p=.0009), and ethnicity (B=.16, p=.02) were statistically significant at or below the .05 level. These three variables indicated that African American males (69%) were indeed more likely than Anglo American males (42%) to believe that anti-hypertensive medication was too expensive (Chi square=10.2, df=2, p=.006).

A most unexpected finding regarding the individual's beliefs about hypertension were the informants answers to this question: "Once you became aware that your blood pressure was high, what did you do about it?" A statistically significant number of African American males and females chose a different lay consultation and referral process than did Anglo American males and females (Tables 5.20 and 5.21).

For example, African American males tended to implement a ethno-care therapy (ethnomedical remedies and/or diet regimen) or do "nothing" about their high blood pressure more often than Anglo American males. Anglo American males (33%), on the otherhand, were more likely to seek a physician to treat their high blood pressure than were African American males (10%) (Chi square=13.5, df=4, p=.008).

TABLE 5.20: Treatment Actions: Males

	African Americans		Anglo Americans	
	N	(%)	N	(%)
Health Care Decision				
Physician	7	(10.3%)	8	(33.3%)
Clinic	1	(1.5%)	0	
Folk Regimen	18	(26.5%)	1	(4.2%)
Nothing	42	(62.7%)	15	(62.5%)
	68		24	

Chi Square = 13.5, df = 3, p = 0.008

TABLE 5.21:Treatment Actions: Females

| | African Americans | | Anglo Americans | |
	N	(%)	N	(%)
Health Care Decision				
Physician	20	(19.0%)	18	(31.6%)
Clinic	11	(10.5%)	0	
Folk				
Regimen	43	(41.0%)	8	(14.0%)
Healer	6	(5.7%)	0	
Nothing	25	(23.8%)	31	(54.4%)
	105		57	

Chi Square = 31.3, df = 4, p = .000
Missing cases = 4

A similar relationship was found between African American and Anglo American females. African American females (41%) stated that they were more likely to use an ethno-care therapy than were Anglo American females (14%). African American females also indicated that the clinic (11%) and a "folk" health practitioner would be their choice for consultation and therapy (Table 5.20). Anglo American females (32%) stated that they would seek a physician to treat their high blood pressure more often than did African American females (19%) (Chi square=31.3, df=5, p=.000). The differences in ethno-care therapy between African Americans and Anglo Americans remain significant across income levels

(Tables 5.22 - 5.26). The results from this question show that more African Americans followed a lay or folk consultation/referral and treatment pattern than did Anglo Americans. These differences in treatment action indicate that Anglo Americans rely on the allopathic support system, whereas African Americans tend to rely on the extensive 'lay' support system.

TABLE 5.22: Treatment Actions: Income $5,000 - $9,999

Health Care Decision	African Americans N	(%)	Anglo Americans N	(%)
Physician	4	(10.8%)	5	(50.0%)
Clinic	2	(5.4%)	0	
Folk Regimen	13	(35.1%)	1	(10.0%)
Healer	4	(10.8%)	0	
Nothing	1	(2.7%)	1	(10.0%)
No Answer	13	(35.1%)	3	(30.0%)
	37		10	

Chi Square = 10.6, df = 5, p = .05

TABLE 5.23: Treatment Actions: Income
$10,000 - $14,999

	African Americans		Anglo Americans	
	N	(%)	N	(%)
Health Care Decision				
Physician	6	(15.8%)	5	(45.5%)
Clinic	3	(7.9%)	0	
Folk Regimen	8	(21.1%)	2	(18.2%)
Healer	1	(2.6%)	0	
Nothing	13	(34.2%)	0	
No Answer	7	(18.4%)	4	(36.4%)
	38		11	

Chi Square = 9.5, df = 5, p = .08

TABLE 5.24: Treatment Actions: Income
$15,000 - $24,999

	African Americans		Anglo Americans	
	N	(%)	N	(%)
Health Care Decision				
Physician	7	(16.7%)	5	(35.7%)
Clinic	7	(16.7)	0	
Folk Regimen	13	(31.0%)	0	

Nothing	5	(11.9%)	2	(14.3%)
No Answer	10	(23.8%)	7	(50.0%)
	42		14	

Chi Square = 10.8, df = 4, p = .02

TABLE 5.25: Treatment Actions: Income
$25,000 - $34,999

	African Americans		Anglo Americans	
	N	(%)	N	(%)
Health Care Decision				
Physician	3	(16.7%)	3	(21.4%)
Clinic	1	(5.6%)	0	
Folk Regimen	9	(50.0%)	1	(7.1%)
Nothing	0		3	(21.4%)
No Answer	5	(27.8%)	7	(50.0%)
	18		14	

Chi Square = 10.3, df = 4, p = .03

**TABLE 5.26: Treatment Actions: Income
$35,000 or More**

	African Americans		Anglo Americans	
	N	(%)	N	(%)
Health Care Decision				
Physician	4	(21.1%)	4	(25.0%)
Folk Regimen	7	(36.8%)	2	(12.5%)
No Answer	8	(42.1%)	10	(62.5%)
	19		16	

Chi Square = 2.7, df = 2, p = .2
*10 African Americans - No Answer to Income Level
*14 Anglo Americans - No Answer to Income Level
** Total Missing Cases = 15

Demographics and Blood Pressure

A multiple regression analysis indicated that a number of variables contributed to the variance in systolic and diastolic blood pressure levels (Tables 5.27 and 5.28 - see appendix). The set of variables, interacting together, explained or accounted for 25% of the variation of the samples' systolic blood pressure, leaving 75% of the variation unexplained. The variables that follow were tested because they have been documented to exhibit a relationship with blood pressure (Dawber et al. 1967; Henry and Cassel 1969; Page 1974 and 1980). Of the 12 variables, 5 were significant at the .05 level: Being diagnosed hypertensive (B=.28, p=.000), Educational Level (B=-.16, p=.01), Unemployed (B=.17, p=.007), Acknowledging perceived symptoms (B=-.16, p=.01), and Age (B=.14, p=.04).

For diastolic blood pressure, the 14 variables accounted for 26% of the total variance. Significant variables included state anxiety (B=.18, p=.01), Diagnosed Hypertensive (B=-.24, p=.000), Family History of HBP (B=-.13, p=.04), Salted Food (B=-.17, p=.01) and Age (B=.16, p=.03).

Nevertheless, a Pearson correlation found that education and state anxiety were only slightly correlated with systolic and diastolic blood pressures. The informants' educational level had an inverse relationship with both systolic (r=-.23, p=.000) and diastolic (r=-.16, p=.01) blood pressures. As an individual's educational level decreased, his/her blood pressure tended to increase. State anxiety, a psychosocial variable, showed a positive correlation with both systolic (r=.16, p=.0006) and diastolic (r=.23, p=.000) blood pressures. Hence, as the individual's anxiety level increased, blood pressure also increased.

Psychosocial Stress: State Anxiety

Of the nine variables interacting in the multiple regression analyses, 3 were statistically significant. These variables were: sex (B=-.39, p=.00), ethnicity (B=-.14, p=.02), and unemployment (B=.21, p=.00). Other variables approaching significance were education (B=-.12, p=.06), age (B=-.11, p=.08), and number of children (B=-.11, p=.07).

A closer examination of the variables in question shows the differences in mean anxiety scores between several groups. Mean state anxiety for the population was 31.0 (SD=8.2).

State anxiety scores for males (39.3, SD=13.1) were significantly higher than females (27.9, SD=7.9, t=8.52, df=247, p=.000). In addition, mean state anxiety for African Americans (34.1, SD=12.6) was significantly higher than for Anglo Americans (27.5, SD=7.0, t=4.22, df=248, p=.000). Mean anxiety scores also differentiated between groups based on their employment and marital status and their age. For instance, unemployment informants had significantly higher mean state anxiety scores (37.5, SD=12.8) than did employed informants (30.5, SD=10.7, t=4.13, df=248, p=.000). Secondly, a one-way analysis (ANOVA) revealed that individuals who were either single (35.5, SD=12.7) or married (32.8, SD=11.8) had significantly higher anxiety scores than those who were widowed informants (26.5, SD=5.2, p=.05). Mean state anxiety score for divorced informants was 29.2 (SD=10.1). In addition, informants who identified their occupation as clerical or sales (40.7, SD=13.1) or who were in skilled trades (41.4, SD=14.4) scored significantly higher mean anxiety scores (p=.05) than did professional workers (25.4, SD=4.7), managers (29.3, SD=11.2), houseworkers (28.9, SD=7.6), and retirees (28.4, SD=9.1). Finally, informants in the 18-34 yr.-age group had significantly higher anxiety scores (36.6, SD=12.3) than those in the 56-90 yr.-age group (29.1, SD=9.1, p=.05).

Pearson correlations identified other sociodemographic variables related to state anxiety. Total family income (r=-.16, p=.01) and educational level (r=-.16, p=.01) were negatively associated (weak) with mean state anxiety scores.

Utilization of Health Screening

A majority of the informants (54%) stated that they had previously attended a Health-O-Rama screening. Despite this promising percentage, a large disparity existed between ethnic groups. African Americans, for example, were significantly less likely than Anglo Americans to have been participants of Health-O-Rama. Only 28 percent of African American males attended a Health-O-Rama screening before compared to 79 percent for Anglo American males. A lower percentage of African American females (52%) had been participants of Health-O-Rama than Anglo American females (74%) (Chi square=6.4, df=1, p=.01).

Table 5.29 shows that age (B=-.22, p=.00), sex (B=-.13, p=.03), and ethnicity (B=-.21, p=.002) were statistically significant. Perceived symptoms almost reached statistical significance in the multiple regression analysis (B=-.11, p=.07). These variables suggest that age, sex, ethnicity, and an individual's perceived symptoms of high blood pressure influenced the informants participation in the health screenings.

Table 5.29: Health Screening Participation

Independent Variables	Beta	t	p=
Unemployed	.02	.36	.71
Family History BP	.00	.12	.90
Age	-.23	-3.50	.00*
Perceived Symptom	-.11	-1.75	.07
Education	-.08	-1.22	.22

Sex	-.13	-2.11	.03*
Ethnicity	-.20	-3.01	.00*
Occupation	.08	1.29	.27
Family			
Income	-.07	-1.09	.27

```
Multiple R = .43
R square   = .19        *Significant Variables
Adjusted R = .16
Standard   = .46
  error
```

Informants were then asked, "Why did you come to the screening today?" The answers to this question supplied suggestions regarding ethnic differences in the level of lay consultation and referral. African American and Anglo American females exhibited statistically significant differences. African American females stated that family members or friends (11%) and perceived symptoms (8%) influenced their decision to participate in the screening; whereas Anglo American females (47%) attended the health screening primarily to check their physician's blood pressure readings. A significant percentage of Anglo American females (19%) also indicated that they had visited the hospital or a physician for an illness 10 or more times within the past year.

Since African American informants appeared to rely more on the extensive 'lay' network for treatment actions than Anglo American informants, a multiple regression analysis examined which factors contributed the most variance to an individual's reasons for not seeking a physician's care when he or she should have. Table 5.30 shows that the nine variables in question explained 21% of the variance.

Informants were asked, "Have you not sought health care when you should have?" Sixty-six percent of African American males and 45% of African American females answered "yes" compared to 29% of Anglo American males and 26% of Anglo American females (Chi square=8.4, df=1, p=.003, Chi square=4.8, df=1, p=.02). This response as well as the qualitative data from the 1986 Health Screening suggest that Detroit African Americans' health care seeking pattern differed from that of Anglo Americans and that this behavior is significantly influenced by sociodemographic, psychosocial, and ethnomedical factors.

Table 5.30: Not Seek Physician Care

Independent Variables	Beta	t	p=
Unemployed	-.22	-3.51	.005*
Family History BP	.14	2.47	.01*
Age	.18	2.90	.004*
Perceived Symptom	.15	2.55	.01*
Education	.15	2.28	.02*
Sex	.13	2.24	.02*
Ethnicity	.17	2.61	.009*
Occupation	.01	.09	.92
Family Income	.15	2.26	.02*

Multiple R   = .46
R square   = .22   *Significant Variables
Adjusted R   = .18
Standard   = .44
 error

CONCLUSION

The 1985 health survey of 82 African Americans and 96 Anglo Americans found that age and income level contributed the most variance to an individual's systolic blood pressure level. Although there were no significant correlation between blood pressure level and state anxiety scores, the relationship was in the direction expected (p=.15). Sociodemographic factors such as being unemployed and a low income level, nonetheless, contributed to an individual's heightened stress level.

The 1985 study also found that the only health belief indice which influenced utilization of health screening was perceived costs. With regard to treatment therapy for anti-hypertensive medication, financial cost was extremely important. In particular, more African Americans than Anglo Americans stated that blood pressure medication was indeed expensive. The 1985 findings, therefore, highlighted the effects of sociodemographic factors and ethnomedical beliefs upon an individual's health care seeking pattern.

The quantitative data from the 1986 health screenings supplied additional information regarding: (1) the sociodemographic and psychosocial factors that affected an individual's blood pressure; and (2) the sociocultural and psychosocial factors which influenced the health care seeking pattern among Detroit African Americans. The findings from 176 African Americans and 82 Anglo Americans showed that factors such as age, family history of high blood pressure, being diagnosed hypertensive, adding salt to foods, unemployment, degree of education, and anxiety level contributed to the variance in systolic and diastolic blood pressure levels. Significant differences in blood pressure did not occur between African Americans and Anglo Americans. Unlike the 1985 findings, the 1986 quantitative data revealed that age, sex, ethnicity, and an individual's perceived symptoms of high blood pressure influenced the informants participation in the health screening. In particular, African Americans tended to rely more on the extensive "lay" network for treatment actions than Anglo Americans. To treat high blood pressure, African Americans often used "folk" or "personal" care treatment therapies prior to medical consultation with mainstream health care practitioners. The 1986 and 1985 quantitative analyses, therefore, support the hypothesis that African Americans exhibit a different health care seeking pattern to Anglo Americans.

Chapter 6

HEALTH CARE SEEKING PATTERNS: A QUALITA-
TIVE ANALYSIS

INTRODUCTION

Although the quantitative findings from the 1985 and 1986 health screenings provided substantial information, the qualitative research (ethnographic data) yielded additional insights about the participants lifestyles and health care seeking pattern. The informal interviews, individual health profiles, and observations conducted during and after the 1986 health screenings form the basis of this segment of the study. Thus, the use of relatively unstructured and semi-structured interviews (Health Belief and Spielberger's State Anxiety Questionnaires) in conjunction with the key informant interviews supported the validity and reliability of the findings of this study.

To analyze the qualitative data of Detroit African Americans, I used thematic and pattern analyses which identifies and brings together components or fragments of ideas or experiences which are often meaningless when viewed alone. While thematic and pattern analyses are closely related, they are not precisely the same. Patterns are generally small units of behavior that contribute to themes. Themes are large units of analysis derived from patterns which can explain multiple aspects of human behavior (Leininger 1985:61).

In studying the health care seeking pattern of Detroit African Americans with regard to hypertension, I discovered five themes: (1) degree of activity and responsibility, (2) individual and familial moral strength, (3) naturalistic causation, (4) family, folk, or personal care, and (5) physical and spiritual balance. This chapter examines the components of the health care seeking process among Detroit African Americans as well as their health and illness beliefs (ethnohealth) and treatment therapies (ethnotherapy) concerning hypertension.

ETHNOHEALTH

As stated in Chapter Two, African American ethnomedical beliefs and practices are a composite, containing elements from a variety of sources: European folklore, Greek classical medicine, modern scientific medicine, and particularly African folklore. These diverse threads are tied together by the tenets of fundamentalist Christianity, elements from the Voodoo religion, and the added spice of sympathetic magic (Snow 1977). It should be emphasized that this health belief system is not exclusively confined to African Americans but also shared by segments of the Anglo American population. By analyzing the health care seeking pattern among Detroit African Americans, we can learn much about their heatlth care practices as well as something of the health care practices of other ethnic groups in the United States.

HEALTH CARE SEEKING BEHAVIOR

Health care behavior is a concept which describes the events that take place when a person is sick. This behavioral pattern includes steps taken by an individual who perceives a need for help as he or she attempts to solve a health problem (Chrisman 1977:353). These steps are conceptually differentiated as elements in the health care seeking process: (1) symptom definition (2) illness-related shifts in role behavior, (3) lay consultation and referral, (4) treatment actions, and (5) adherence. As health care researchers, however, we must understand the individual's concept of "health" and "illness" before appropriate treatment is suggested.

DETROIT AFRICAN AMERICAN HEALTH CARE PATTERNS

Health
Health refers to the beliefs, values, and action-patterns that are culturally known and are used to preserve and maintain personal or group well-being, and to perform daily activities; whereas ethnohealth refers to the individual's beliefs and patterns (emic) concerning preventative health care (Leininger 1985:196). The importance of distinguishing these two concepts helps delineate the difference between the cultural and ethnic acceptance of what constitutes "being healthy."

For example, the following typified my general informants' response to the question, "What does being healthy mean to you?:

Healthy means being able to live day by day.
Healthy is doin' whatever I have to do to stay alive.
Health is just livin'.
Health is bein' able to run with the boys.
Healthy means exercising regularly.
Healthy means watching weight, diet, exercise, and
caring for my family.

The preceeding responses indicate that "being healthy" encompasses a degree of activity and responsibility.

Some general informants perceived health as a day-to-day personal event with little activity required; while to others health consisted of being able to participate in day-to-day familial or social events with a relatively high level of activity and responsibility. Obviously cultural variables affect the informants definition of health, as the degree of activity and responsibility are related to such cultural values as individual and familial strength, an emphasis on present orientation, and survival of the family. Harrison and Harrison (1971), Hines (1972), Orque et al. (1983), Leininger (1985), Manuel (1986), and Sussman et al. (1987) have found similar definitions of health among other samples of African Americans. Since general and key informants have a broad perspective of what constitutes "being healthy," they also have a different perception of what constitutes an "illness."

Illness
Illness-causing agents derive from two etiological principles -- naturalistic and personalistic. Naturalistic causation beliefs identify impersonal internal or external agents which interact

to produce illness. Such impersonal agents as microbes, inadequate rest, poor nutrition, accidents, environmental pol-
lutants, as well as beliefs about imbalances in hot, cold, dry,
and moist bodily humors, or disharmony between the positive
and negative forces determine what caused an illness.

  Personalistic causation beliefs identify personal agents as
culprits of illness. These agents may be either spiritual en-
titites (ghost, souls, deities, or devils) or human agents
(witches, shamans, or priests) who have extraordinary powers
to cause illness and/or health. Thus here the major factor is
not what, but who, caused an illness (Chino and Vollweiler
1986:245). In this sample of Detroit African Americans'
etiological beliefs of hypertension, ninety-seven percent identified naturalistic agents as the primary cause of their illness.
General and key informants considered inadequate rest, poor
nutrition, weather disturbances, and imbalances in hot and
cold properties as naturalistic agents affecting their blood
pressure. For instance, Willie, a 56 year-old African
American male, believed that an individual's blood viscosity
is directly related to the weather and one's age. This informant stated, "my blood is probably high today because it's a little chilly outside and I'm gettin' older." Furthermore, Mr.
King, a 62 year-old, middle income African American male,
felt that he became susceptible to high blood pressure
primarily because of his active daily lifestyle. The informant
stated, "if you stay out too long or are too active, then that is
the cause of your illness." Thus, ethnomedical beliefs regarding high blood pressure related to their general definition of
illness: "Disharmony with nature."

Symptom Definition of High Blood Pressure

An individual's symptom definition develops when the degree of discomfort becomes noticeable and acknowledgeable by his/her cultural group. If the illness receives a "cultural stamp," then, a health care action follows (Chrisman 1986:2). Yet, how can an individual formulate his/her symptom definition of an illness if there are usually no symptoms associated with the illness as in the case of essential hypertension? From a medically-orthodox perspective, essential hypertension is a cardiovascular disease of unknown origin. The most perplexing attribute of essential hypertension is that - according to the medical profession - there are usually no symptoms associated with it -- that it is asymptomatic. According to hypertension health professionals, a person cannot tell what his/her blood pressure's by how he/she feels. The only way to know one's pressure is to have it measured.

Most people, however, are unaccustomed to thinking about high blood pressure in asymptomatic terms because symptoms often provide the starting point for speculations about illness. A majority of the sampled Detroit African Americans (63%) perceived such syptoms as headaches, dizziness, tenseness, dry lips, seeing spots, and ringing in ears associated with their elevated blood pressure. These symptoms helped to formulate their symptom definition of hypertension plus beliefs about "high blood" and "low blood."

In addition, a majority of my informants (80%) did not feel that the degree of discomfort from the perceived symptoms warrented a health action. From this perspective one's illness can be perceived as "ill-at-ease -- a state of disease" without being functionally incapacitated (Jacques 1976:121).

Illness Related Shifts in Role Behavior
Since all cultural and ethnic groups associate modified rights and obligations with the "sick role," the ill person is often not separated from all the responsibilities of his familiar environment. Informants who had been previously diagnosed as hypertensive continued their role responsibilities. Even among the more severe cases, individuals maintained their daily activities. When asked, "What are the chief problems your illness/symptom has caused you?", eighty percent replied "absolutely nothing" or "it only lasted a few minutes." Since hypertension (mild and sometimes severe) was not perceived as a serious illness, informants retained most of their role obligations by modifying daily activities.

Lay Consultation and Referral
The lay consultation and referral relate specifically to the patterns of choice among potential consultants and the content of consultants' responses to the sick individual. Those who share similar health beliefs and practices and social networks of the sick individual obviously have a direct impact on the "type" of health care received. The patterns of lay consultation and referral among Detroit African Americans, particularly the elderly, illustrate how the extensive social network influenced their health care seeking behavior.

For example, a high-income normotensive African American female associated her severe headaches with a gradual elevation of blood pressure. Although the severe headaches persisted for days, she sought much of her medical advice from immediate family members -- aunt and mother. Another African American female (middle-aged, slightly-overweight and normotensive) traveled from Grand Rapids, MI. (148 miles) to participate in the free health screening on the advice from Detroit relatives. Informants, therefore, trusted and followed the advice of friends and extended family members before attending or avoiding available health services.

The reasons why Detroit African Americans (11% females and 16% males), as well as other ethnic groups, used their informal lay network extensively for medical problems was primarily because: (1) the reciprocal give-and-take relationships between the individual and family, friends, extended non-kin members can act as a buffer between the individual and the stressful situation; (2) such interactions helps the person to cope better with the situation either instrumentally or psychologically, and because (3) such contacts set the stage for facing the need to go to professional health care providers to get treatment and medication. Thus, a person employing such a treatment action may redefine the situation as being not stressful (or as being less stressful), may try to think out alternative ways to deal with the situation, may evaluate the consequences of different actions, or may employ a variety of other cognitive strategies.

Treatment Actions

Tables 5.20 and 5.26 show that African Americans and Anglo Americans exhibited significant differences in the type of treatment sought and source of treatment advice (see Chapter 5). General informants were asked, "Once you became aware that your blood pressure was high, what did you do about it?" African American males were more likely than Anglo American males to implement a personal or family 'folk' care regimen (26.5% - 4.2%) or do 'nothing' (23.5% - 8.3%) when they became aware that their blood pressure was elevated. Similarly, African American females were more likely than Anglo American females to use a folk care regimen (41% - 14%) to seek treatment from a clinic (10.5% - 0%), and to consult a healer (5.7% - 0%) for their elevated blood pressure level.

The differences between African Americans' and Anglo Americans' choice of treatment actions reflected socioeconomic constraints as well as adherence to ethnomedical beliefs and practices. The adherence to these ethnomedical practices helps African Americans to cope better with the perceived illness both instrumentally and psychologically (spiritually); thereby redefining the situation as less stressful and less serious.

Ethno-Care

The types and sources of treatment actions among Detroit informants varied according to socioeconomic status and degree of assimilation to mainstream society. Since a majority of the elderly Detroit African Americans (approximately

70%) are first generation Southern migrants, my sample tended to use home remedies and nonprescribed (patent) medicines suggested to them by their lay network. Of the 176 informants, 43 (41%) females and 18 (27%) males implemented a ethno-care therapy. The following cases typify my informants response to high blood pressure.

Informant 1:

A 54 year-old African American woman, who migrated to Detroit in the late 1940s, stated that there are certain illnesses a person must "live with."

Because of her low income and a good rapport with an elderly physician, this woman continued her folk care regimen by following the meal with a pinch of garlic to treat her high blood pressure. The woman's physician, also a southern migrant, suggested the folk care regimen. She attended the health screening only after her perceived symptoms associated with high blood pressure became too serious to neglect.

Informant 3:

A 35 year-old health professional African American male sought advice primarily from his mother. Because this individual felt that he is "in-tune" with his body and because his mother never sought physician's care (use of folk remedies), he stated, "I will seek a physician's care only as a last resort."

Informant 4:

A 59 year-old African American woman who practices a folk care regimen (vinegar and herbal teas) to treat her high blood pressure, believes that one's health is the responsibility of the individual, not the physician Moreover, her lack of information about the seriousness of high blood pressure and the hereditary component of hypertension had delayed her from seeking health care from medically trained professionals.

Informant 6:

A 73 year-old African American woman who believes that African Americans need more education about health care practices; she stated, "we are raised not to question the doctor even if the information is not totally understood" (Bailey 1987)

Informant 24:

A 43 year-old high-income African American female (administrator) perceived a number of symptoms with her elevated blood pressure. Her treatment involved self-diagnosis of daily activities and implementing lifestyle modifications.

Informant 54:

A middle-aged African American man with a history of essential hypertension who uses sassafras and leaf teas in treating his slightly elevated blood pressure; although under doctor's care, he continues his folk treatment regimen in conjunction with his physician's prescribed medication because, "If I tell him that I am using herbs, he would think that I was silly" (Bailey 1988:1110).

Informant 67:
An elderly African American hypertensive female who perceived symptoms with high blood pressure took epsom salt and cream of tartar to thin her blood. She stated that it is important for the individual to use the proper amounts since excessive proportions of these home remedies may lower one's blood pressure too far (thin blood).

The preceeding informants showed that personal or family folk treatment regimens for high blood pressure varied from altering one's activity to consuming such astringent substances as epsom salts, sassafras teas, garlic tablets, vinegar, lemon juice, asprins, and cream of tartar (Table 6.1). Informants indicated that not only did these astringent substances lower their blood pressure but also flushed the body of all impurities. Moreover, regardless of the type of home remedy or patent medicine used by the informant, self-prescribed home medications were generally taken prior to medical consultations and continued after consultation with prescribed medications, even though the informant did not tell the physician of this fact.

**Table 6.1: Types of Ethnomedical Remedies
for High Blood Pressure**

Type	Number Identified
Epsom Salt	15
Garlic Tablets	14
Sassafras Tea	2
Vinegar	2
Lemon Juice	2
Cream of Tartar	2
Leaf Tea	2
Diet (reducing salt, cholesterol, 'richy' foods or activity	37
Water	3
Celery	1
Catnip Tea	1
Aspirin	1

Sample: 41%(43) African American Females and
27%(18) African American Males

*Informants   used   1   or   several   ethnomedical
remedies.

Alternative or Folk Health Practitioners

There are a variety of alternative or folk health practitioners serving the African American community. The four types of African American alternative/folk healers are: (1) independent generalists (2) independent specialists, (3) cultic generalists, and (4) cultic specialists. Eleven percent of the female informants consulted the independent specialist to treat their high blood pressure.

Independent specialists are mainly herbalists, neighborhood prophets, and magic store vendors. Each specialist has the capacity to treat a wide variety of physical and mental problems. Like traditional African folk healers, these African American alternative/folk practitioners use treatments such as religious rituals, herbs and roots, and the observance of certain prohibitions or directions to cure individuals (Baer 1985, Goodson 1987, Hill 1976, Jordan 1979, and Tinling 1967). Probably the best known independent specialist is the herbalist.

I visited four herbalist establishments in the Detroit Metropolitan area, as suggested by my informants. Such alternative/folk health practitioners as herbalist and magic store vendors dispensed medicines for a wide range of prices. Treatment therapy consists usually of dandelion and valerian root, or garlic tablets and garlic supplements or advice to reduce salt, fatty foods, and stress. Although the alternative/folk health practitioners had various ideas about the promptness of the prescribed herbs in lower one's blood pressure, they did agree, on the effectivness of their remedies.

The basic assumption behind the use of herbs links the natural organic properties of herbs with the natural healing capabilities of man. Herbalists use these organic substances in an effort to neutralize or eliminate one's body of harmful substances that impair its power to heal itself (Lust 1974:8). According to herbalists, any herb if mixed and used properly can treat effectively any natural illness.

The reasons why my informants consulted the various alternative/folk health practitioners for treating their high blood pressure were: (1) their attempt to cope with health problems within the context of their own resources and social environment; (2) their belief that alternative/folk health practitioners have some control over the forces that cause anomalies in a person's life, whereas westernized medical physicians (mainstream practitioners) cannot heal certain cases of illness and misfortune; and (3) lower monetary expense associated with such treatments.

The purpose of specifying the types of alternative/folk health practitioners used by Detroit African Americans is to illustrate the adaptability, the secretiveness of their herbal concoctions (amount and cost), and the diversity of these skilled specialists. These specialists are not only accepted by the African American community, but are also consulted by the members of the larger society (Baer 1985).

Mainstream Health Practitioners

Although a notable percentage (41% female and 27% male) of my sample of Detroit African Americans used various sources for treatment, other informants (19% female and 10% male) visited mainstream health practitioners. Most of these encounters with health professionals occurred in outpatient or emergency room facilities. The major reasons are:

1. The flight of private office-based physician from inner-city areas during a time when Medicare and Medicaid increased demand (by decreasing financial access barriers) for health services among the elderly and urban poor;

2. The general tendency for the poor and African Americans not to have a regular family physician;

3. The perception among some residents of medically under-served areas that hospitals provide a higher quality of medical care than neighborhood health centers;

4. The tendency of health insurance plans to provide reim-bursement for hospital visits only; and

5. The tradition of free care within hospitals which over the years may have taught many low income people to rely on hospitals as an inexpensive source of medical care.(Neigh-bors 1986:275)

For instance, Florence, a 59 year-old middle-income African American woman, used the outpatient services of a local hospital for treating her hypertension over a 7 year period. During this time period, she has not had the same physician for any extended period of time. This informant indicated that she was extremly satisfied with care received from the various physicians and also that she trusted their judgement. The reason for following an anti-hypertensive regimen and the major factors contributing to her high blood pressure, however, were never explained thoroughly to her. In fact, she asked this researcher what factors contribute to an elevated blood pressure level. Hence, the major health issue concern-ing the Detroit sample focused upon the quality of health care received at these mainstream health care facilities. The dif-ficulty some informants had of understanding the medical ex-planation of physicians and their inability to participate actively in the discussion of their illness affected not only the quality of care but also their adherence to prescribed treatment regimens.

Adherence
The final step of the health care seeking process, adherence, refers to the degree to which the sick person acts upon the treatment advice. The cases which follow show various forms of adherence to the indivdual's preventative health care regimen and/or mainstream health care regimen.

Ms. Lester, a 44 year-old, middle income, African American health care professional, adhered to a folk ethnomedical treatment pattern as well as the mainstream treatment pattern. As a native Detroiter, this woman received her medical training from a local university and thereafter served as a nurse clinician for ten years at a major urban hospital. She eventually became disenchanted with the clinical aspect of the medical field, and switched to the health insurance field because she felt that it would better serve the African American community primarily.

As a divorced parent, this informant was assisted by her extended family network in raising her two children; her parents, brothers, sisters, and great aunt all assisted in the care of her children. Although she received training and worked in mainstream health care facilities for 20 years, she often sought advice for treating minor and serious illnesses from extended familial members. For instance, symptoms associated with high blood pressure (headaches, blurred vision, and throbbing pain) were treated with white potatoes around the back of the neck and eyes in an effort to absorb the pain. If the pain persisted, aspirin and leaf tea were taken in varying amounts. This informant learned and adhered to these treatment remedies from her training in the medical field but from her great aunt and the local folk practitioner.

The case of another woman, typifies a majority of my informants' responses to severe hypertension. Raised as a responsible and health care oriented individual, this informant became a highly prestigious informal leader within the community. Her 30 years of services to the community established Mrs. Johnson as a spokesperson for the elderly. In fact, she organized a majority of the social and health care activities for the local senior citizens group. Although this woman was quite astute as to mainstream preventive health care practices, she experienced some difficulties in adhering to such patterns.

Diagnosed with borderline hypertension in her thirties, this elderly woman attempted to adhere stringently to the anti-hypertensive regimen prescribed by her physician. During the past 33 years, however, her blood pressure has increased steadily (currently 160/90 mmHg); thereby causing her to question the physician's anti-hypertensive therapy. Although her physician suggested a number of behavioral modifications, the informants' non-awareness of the risk factors associated with hypertensives (family history, cholesterol level, and obesity) and the financial, logistic, and ethnically influenced inability) to make the adjustments to mainstream health care patterns allowed her to discredit the efficacy of the treatment therapy and search for other means (ethnomedical remedies) to control her blood pressure. This informant emphasized frequently that as a senior citizen she simply does not have the time or energy to make the type of behavior modifications which her doctor requested. As she stated, "I'm in charge of 40 - 50 senior citizens who can barely take care of themselves." "How can I afford the time and money to look for the things that my doctor said." "I have too many people depending on me just to survive." "Besides my herbs and teas have been doin' me just fine."

To understand how the total array of sociocultural and ethnohistorical factors influence an individual's ethnomedical beliefs and treatment pattern for high blood pressure, the following two cases are presented. The first, a 56-year old African American man, left Mississippi at age nine and went to Chicago where his uncle resided. Incorporated into his uncle's family, he earned his stay with odd jobs for 9 years. When he reached 18, this man immediately enlisted into the service. Although he had fond memories of the army, he indicated that on many occasions he had to defend himself and other Black soldiers from the hostility of the White service men.

After his years in the service, this returned to Chicago for two years and then moved to Detroit where his sister lived. As a landscape laborer, he worked 14 years for his sister's construction company. He later acquired a job at the Chrysler plant, and worked on the assembly line for seven years before retiring due to multiple health disorders (liver, kidney, and high blood pressure).

Despite the efforts of this man's wife and physician to modify his dietary and lifestyle pattern, he considers himself quite "healthy." Because he can get up and walk around the community to socialize with his friends on a daily basis, he perceives high blood pressure (illness) as "ill-at-ease - a state of disease" without his being functionally incapacitated. In addition, he rationalizes that his blood was probably high primarily because of the cold temperature outside; old age also increases one's blood thickness (Bailey 1988:1110). To lower his blood pressure, he would use his wife's medication periodically, as well as small portions of alcohol to thin his blood. This man's ethnomedical beliefs regarding high blood pressure related to his general definition of health and illness and his perceived low status in society. He says his condition results from, "Disharmony with nature and disharmony with society's standards."

Finally, Harold a 68 year-old hypertensive African American man shows how a conservative gentleman integrated the physician's treatment regimen into his ethnomedical belief system for controlling his blood pressure. Originally a resident of a small town in Alabama, this informant migrated in 1953, seeking better paying jobs in northern cities. Upon arrival in Detroit, he found a job at one of the auto plants and lived in the Grand Boulevard area with his wife. Once settled, they sought health care primarily at one of the large urban hospitals. After selecting a primary physician, both were diagnosed with mild hypertension. As the years passed, the Boulevard became too expensive, and in 1978 the couple moved to one of the public housing complexes in the

City of Detroit. This informant experienced some trying times in this neighborhood. First, his wife of 40 years died of a heart attack. His wife's physician suggested that if he did not change his lifestyle, he would meet the same fate as his wife. When this traumatic experience was coupled with the change in the neighborhood (slightly higher crime rate), this man found it extremely difficult to adapt to the problems of everyday life and particularly of adhering to the physician's treatment regimen.

Nonetheless, since this informant's beliefs in naturalistic causation acknowledged that one's blood is affected by such "richy" foods as heavily salted greens, pork, and sweets, he found that modifying his diet in accordance with the physician's suggestions was not as difficult as he had originally thought. Moreover, the help he received from the senior citizens' group provided additional psychological and spiritual support in following the physician's therapy. This man commented, "I didn't know that I could continue eatin' my good home cooked meals and still be followin' the doctor's orders." Currently, he continues his ethnocare treatment regimen while also adhering to the physician's anti-hypertensive drug treatment regimen.

Tables 6.2 and 6.3 show the use of prescribed anti-hypertensive treatment between African Americans and Anglo Americans.

Table 6.2: Use of Prescribed Anti-Hypertensive Treatment:
Males

	African American		Anglo Americans	
	N	(%)	N	(%)
Yes	17	(25.0%)	8	(33.3%)
No	23	(33.8%)	3	(12.5%)
DK*	3	(4.4%)	11	(25.8%)
DNA*	25	(36.8%)	2	(8.3%)
	—		—	
	68		24	

Chi Square = 28.1, df = 3, p = .000
*DK= Don't Know
*DNA= Did not Answer

Table 6.3: Use of Prescribed Anti-Hypertensive Treatment:
Females

	African American		Anglo Americans	
	N	(%)	N	(%)
Yes	30	(28.6%)	28	(48.3%)
No	21	(20.0%)	10	(17.2%)
DK*	32	(30.5%)	17	(29.3%)
DNA*	22	(21.0%)	3	(5.2%)
	—		—	
	105		58	

```
Chi Square = 10.3, df = 3, p = .01
Missing Cases = 3
*DK= Don't Know
*DNA= Did not Answer
```

In this case, the informant realized the "chronicity" and "seriousness" of hypertension. Yet for many of my informants, hypertension was believed to be a "curable" illness, one which the individual can self-treat. This belief in naturalistic causation reinforced the individual's perception that hypertension was only a minor health problem. But, this minor health problem, if not controlled, inevitably results in serious health consequences.

Once perceived as a serious illness, other informants (95%) searched for a personalistic agent (often God) to help them treat this unforseeable and undectable illness. While continuing their ethno-care regimen, informants included prayers (either alone or with a church leader) as a direct appeal to God in an attempt to cure their illness. Both methods were an effort to restore one's body to harmony with nature: spiritually and biologically.

Thus to summarize, the qualitative analyses revealed the following themes concerning the informants' symptom definition of high blood pressure: (1) cultural definition of being 'healthy,' (2) naturalistic or personalistic causation of illness, (3) perceived severity of symptoms (acuteness and duration), and (4) health beliefs of 'lay' network. In addition, the decisive factors in the utilization or non-utilization of the health screening were: (1) perceived costs, (2) perceived efficacy of treatment, (3) perceived severity of symptoms (acute vs chronic), (4) perceived cues to action (internal and/or external), (5) health beliefs of 'lay' network, (6) type of health facility (mall vs community health center or church), (7) southern migrant, and (8) adherence to traditional African American cultural beliefs such as importance of spiritualism, emphasis on the present, trust, strong authority structure, admiration to older adults, and individual and familial moral strength.

Finally, from the informal and semi-structured interviews, individual health profiles, and direct observations, the following outline profiles the health care seeking pattern and the resources utilized among the sampled Detroit African Americans.

Profile of Health Care Seeking Steps Among Detroit African Americans

1. Illness appears (perceived symptoms associated with high blood pressure);

2. Individual waits for a certain period (delays days or weeks);

3. Allows body to heal itself (prayer or ethno-medical regimens);

4. Diagnoses daily activities (reduce work or stress);

5. Seeks advice from family member or close friend (church leader and/or alternative health practitioner included; and

6. Attends health screening clinic or family physician.

Resources Utilized

1. Ethnomedical ethno-care remedies (sassafras tea, garlic tablets, epsom salt, vinegar, lemon juice, cream of tartar, water, catnip tea, and celery)

2. Mainstream ethno-care remedies (aspirin and anti-hypertensive medication)

3. Ethnomedical health care practices (natural healing properties of the body, reduce "richy" foods, and environmental stressors)

4. Mainstream health care practices (reduce sodium cholesterol and stress, and increase exercise)

5. Alternative/folk healers (respected elderly family member or friend, herbalist, spiritualist, magic store vendor, evangelistic healer , and the Lord)

6. Mainstream practitioners (pharmacists, outpatient physicians, nurses, and family physician)

Once we recognized the multitude of factors that affect health care seeking behavior among African American patients, utilization and adherence to mainstream health care facilities should improve.

CONCLUSION

This review of the health care seeking process examined how health beliefs and practices affected the degree of interaction with various health practitioners. The ethnic and social bond an individual may develop toward his/her health beliefs and practices clearly helps African Americans to cope better with an illness either objectively or spiritually.

Despite its seeming inclusiveness, the health care seeking process is a basis in constructing theories to account for the diversity of health-related behaviors in a complex society. The practical implications of this process enable health professionals to analyze an individual's ethnomedical beliefs and practices concerning a specific illness for the purpose of developing public health intervention strategies which have a positive impact on the health status of the individual as well as on the relevant ethnic population.

Chapter 7

INTERVENTION STRATEGIES FOR URBAN AFRICAN AMERICANS

INTRODUCTION

Community health screening programs were originally designed: (1) to stimulate change in family and community knowledge and behavior relating to the prevention of disease; (2) to inform the use of available health resources; and (3) to improve the environmental, economic, and educational factors related to health (Geiger 1972). Since their inception during the 1960s and 1970s, however, community health screening programs have primarily used conventional approaches to health improvement. That is, the need is not merely for the provision of more preventative and curative health services or the distribution of services to passive recipients, but for the active involvement of local populations in ways which will preserve or repattern their knowledge, attitudes and motivation concerning major health care issues. Thus, when health care professionals design a culturally-oriented community health screening program, it is intended to address five major issues: (1) to alert a target group to health issues, (2) to help them make choices, (3) to maintain some of their traditional health care practices, (4) to encourage them to try new health care practices, and (5) to in-

131

form them of the most straight forward and effective behavioral alternatives for health promotion.

Presently, we realize that implementing preventative health
care services in any community can improve the health status
of its members. Yet, programs designed specifically for
African Americans are even more effective. Health directors
who have worked extensively with the African American
community suggest: (1) locate health services near prominent
African American institutions, (2) increase African American
health personnel, (3) use local residents in various capacities,
and (4) address the individual's total health care and social
needs (Bloch 1976; Whitehead 1984; Campbell 1979; Braithwaite 1989; and Jones 1986).

DETROIT INTERVENTION STRATEGIES

Since the percentage of African American participants in the
health screenings had declined steadily during the past five
years at the United Health Organization's Project Health-O-
Rama Health Screenings, I recommended the following intervention strategies: (1) utilize more local community leaders;
(2) locate influential informal community leaders; (3) incor-
porate other community services; (4) include worksite screenings; (5) create incentives with local businesses; and (6)
advertise and educate through innovative resources.

At one of the oldest and most well-known churches in
Detroit, additional local community leaders were needed.
Key informants emphasized that leaders such as ministers and
deacons should not only announce the health screening
during the church services but should also participate and

plead with members to take part in the available health services. If congregational members see their minister involved in the program, they are more likely to participate since ministers maintain a high status within the African American community. Churches, whether storefront or elite, must therefore be continually incorporated in the health screenings.

There was an obvious need of including other community services in the program. Another local elite church, for example, made a sincere effort to provide a variety of services to increase clientele. Services such as crime prevention, osteopathic examinations, and senior citizens' support groups were present. African Americans who attended these neighborhood health screenings often expected all their problems to be handled at the same place: social, health, familial, and legal. Perhaps additional services such as employment opportunities, foot care, stress management classes, drug counseling, prenatal information, clothing and food outlets could function as special attractions for the target population.

The remaining church sites visited, however, did not provide any other services during their health screening. In fact, most key informants indicated that the local health screening staff failed to work "with" the local residents -- it only worked "for" them. This difference of working "for" or working "with" the African American community has important psychosocial implications. When African Americans perceive a health service as strictly a "hand-out", they believe that the service is of poor quality and demeaning to the psyche of the individual. This perception caused many African Americans not to participate in the local health screenings.

In addition, local businesses should create special discount incentives for residents who participate in the health screening. When health screenings were located in malls, for example, several local merchants expressed a desire to be a part of the health screening but did not know how. Perhaps a 5 - 10% discount on store items from local merchants (shoe, clothing, or record shop) would not only have provided the extra incentive to increase African American representation of total clients screened but also give the perception that local merchants wanted to work "with" the African American community to improve their health status.

Furthermore, rather than rely completely upon the media to advertise the Health-O-Rama screenings, site coordinators should have disseminated information through the informal networks which already exited within the community. A community leader stated the following:

"Many elderly people have been associated with a particular doctor for several years and will not seek any health care service from another source unless it is suggested by a relative or a close friend. Only by disseminating information through the extensive informal network will the potential clients consider seeking another opinion abut their current health condition."

Additionally, the support of such organizations as the League of Catholic Women, United Community Services, and the Detroit Urban League helped advertise the health screening in the local communities. The data from this study support the idea that the extensive informal network can be a viable resource to broadcast information about the forthcoming health screening.

HOUSTON INTERVENTION STRATEGIES

To assess whether the intervention strategies for the sampled Detroit African Americans were truly effective, this medical anthropologist collaborated with local health officials and residents to design a community health screening program in Houston, Texas. This section discusses the development, the design, and the implementation of this culturally-oriented community health screening program for the local African American population.

Population
From the early 1970s to the 1980s, the city of Houston established itself as the premier city in the sunbelt. The prominence of the city was highlighted by such characteristics as being one of the fastest growing cities in the nation (from 1.74 million in 1970 to 2.4 million in 1980), leading the nation in home construction (over 487,000 housing units were added to the area in the 1970s), and serving as a "magnet" for attracting individuals seeking expanding opportunities. The city's growth rate, however, was associated with a few negative consequences of rapid urbanization.

Specifically, the general problems which Houston currently faces are not unlike those of other urban areas: namely, the problems of inadequate housing, deteriorating inner-city neighborhoods, urban crime, disinvestment and redlining in lower-income areas, high youth and minority unemployment, and the absence of a coherent community development "master plan" for inner-city revitalization (Housing Authority of the City of Houston 1983 and Bullard 1982).

Although predicting future sociodemographic trends are widely divergent, the Houston area is expected to exhibit a slight slow-down in population. Located primarily in Harris County, Houston's population rates for 1980-2000 include continuing negative net migration for the over 64 age-group and decreasing but still positive migration for the 20-34 year-age group. By the year 2000, estimated total population is projected to be 3,215,571 (Anglo = 1,789,260, Blacks = 635,158, Hispanic = 712,124 and Other = 79,029).

While Houston's African American population continue to expand outward to all five wards of the city, the largest African American enclaves are in the Fourth Ward, southwest of downtown around the old Freedmantown neighborhood; in the Third Ward, southeast of downtown; and in the Fifth Ward, northeast of the business. Currently, the Third Ward has supplanted the Fifth and Fourth Wards as the hub of African American social, cultural, and economic life in Houston. In addition to being the financial and business center for Houston's African Americans, the Third Ward serves as a center of African American higher education, with the nation's third largest historically African American university, Texas Southern University, located there; African American mass communications, with the three leading African American Houston newspapers and the three African American owned radio stations; and African American civil rights organizations' headquarters (Bullard).

The major problems that confront Houston's African American community today, including the Third Ward, are poor employment and economic status, a high crime rate, and a substandard of health care services. The African American health care system that developed during the period of segregation has all but disappeared. Of the four African American hospitals still operating in the city, only two, Riverside General Hospital and Charles Drew Hospital are still open (Wintz 1984). In an effort to relieve the problems of available heath care to African Americans and other ethnic populations, the city of Houston's Department of Health and Human Services have expanded their operations of health clinics in the Houston area.

Health Service Areas

The Bureau of Health Planning and the Bureau of Epidemiology have divided Houston into 11 geographic areas called Health Service Areas (HSAs). All areas of the city of Houston are included with the exception of the downtown area (Figure 7). The seven primary HSAs are Northside, Casa de Amigos, Lyons, Magnolia, Riverside, Sunnyside and West End. This clinically-applied research project on which this study is based was located at the Riverside Health clinic.

In 1986, Riverside's population estimate totaled 69,798. Blacks accounted for 77.5% of the population, Whites for 12.9%, Hispanics for 7.5% of the population, and Others for 2.1%. Male comprised 48.2% of the population and females 51.8%.

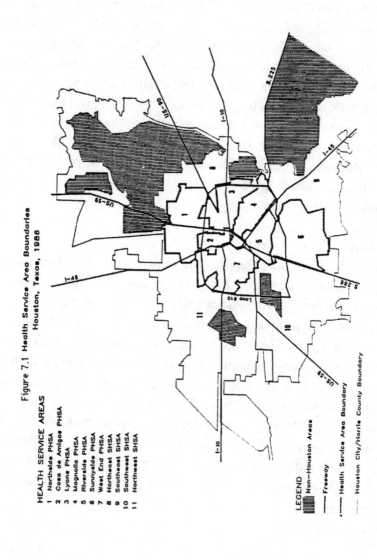

Figure 7.1 Health Service Area Boundaries
Houston, Texas, 1986

HEALTH SERVICE AREAS

1 Northside PHSA
2 Casa de Amigos PHSA
3 Lyons PHSA
4 Magnolia PHSA
5 Riverside PHSA
6 Sunnyside PHSA
7 West End PHSA
8 Northeast SHSA
9 Southeast SHSA
10 Southwest SHSA
11 Northwest SHSA

LEGEND

▨ Non-Houston Areas
━ Freeway
┄ Health Service Area Boundary
┈ Houston City/Harris County Boundary

The average age of the overall population fell within the 25-29 year-age group. The average age of Hispanics and Others was within the 20-24 year-age group. Blacks had an average age within the 25-29 year-age group and Whites had an average age within the 30-34 year-age group.

Socioeconomic indicators listed 24.0% of families as under the poverty level and 36.1% of households as headed by single females. The median household income for 1986 was $15,666.

Method

In order to begin understanding and developing a culturally-oriented health screening program for the local African American community, the principal investigator established a working dialogue and association with three key informants: (1) Shannon Jones (Riverside Health Center Administrator), (2) Dr. Brobbey (Riverside Medical Director), and (3) Mrs. Helen-Hall Kinard (President of Riverside's Advisory Board. The information derived from key informants was primarily gathered through such qualitative techniques as participant observation, casual conversation, semi-structured interviews, and individual life histories (Leininger 1985; Chrisman 1982; and Weidman 1982). These three informants were not only instrumental in the conceptualization and implementation of the community health screening but also of providing substanative qualitative data about Houston Health Department's program procedures and Third Ward residents' needs. Upon requests from the key informants, the principal investigator became a member of Riverside's Advisory Board (1988).

Riverside's Advisory Board mainly consists of local Third Ward residents, Houston Health Department officials, and local businessmen/women. The functions of the Advisory Board entail overseeing the operations of the clinic and developing community programs. Board meetings were held once a month at Riverside Health clinic.

Once the 1989 spring agenda was established, the principal investigator was elected chairman of the 1989 Riverside Health Fair by the Advisory Board. As chairman of the health fair, the principal investigator proposed a modification to the original design of the health fair primarily because the model was outdated and not oriented to the local African American community. The proposed change - to wholistically address the parameters of community health - stimulated much controversy.

Initially, board members considered a "typical" health fair should offer strictly medical services to local residents. Medical services such as cholesterol screening, blood pressure screening, vision screening, and height/weight were the traditional "norm" for a public health fair. Yet after much debate amongst advisory board members, the health fair was finally expanded to include a wide array of health care and social services in an effort to meet the needs of the Third Ward residents. That is, designing a health fair as a "community festival" instead of the typical annual health fair.

In effect, the principal investigator was gradually introducing more awareness of the sociocultural parameters of community health screenings, in a predominantly African American, but culturally diverse community. The principal investigator's advocacy of a "community festival" health fair format was eventually adopted by the Advisory Board due to the support of two informants (President of the Advisory Board and Health Center Administrator) who shared the view that a full range of needs specific to the sociocultural reality of the Riverside community should be served. Selection of the aforementioned tests and services were based upon three criteria: (1) do they address current problems in the community; (2) do they require residents to rely upon African American institutions in the community; and (3) do they help people discover ways to reduce the anxiety and seek health care in the community.

In cooperation with Houston's Department of Health and Human Services and 18 local agencies, basic tests and preventative health services offered at the Riverside Community Health Screening were the following: Height and Weight Screening, Blood Pressure Screening, Vision Screening, Dental Screening, Pulmonary Function Screening, Pre-Natal and Child Care Counseling, Law Enforcement Child Identification Screening, Social Service Counseling, Aids Counseling, and a Aids Education Play. In addition, this one day, free community health screening provided food and prizes to all participants.

Selection of the aforementioned tests and services were based upon three major issues: (1) Addressing the current problems in the community; (2) Utilizing traditional, African American institutions in the community; and (3) Discovering ways to reduce the anxiety of seeking health care in the community.

Results

After 5 months of planning, organizing, and soliciting support from local health care and social agencies, the results of Riverside's 1989 Health Fair was a major success. Since this health screening was the first one-day screening for Riverside Health Clinic, initial projections for total participants was a modest number of 75. Yet final statistics show that over 200 African Americans (participants, providers, and clinic family members) participated in the health screening.

Although the principal investigator was involved with the operations of the community health screening, I noticed that most individuals arrived with several extended familial members belonging to either a young age group (approx. 3-16yrs) or a mature age group (approx. 50-80yrs). It was obvious that individuals who sought health care/social services did so in familial or social/cultural groupings. In addition, the Health Fair was not perceived of as only a "health fair" but as a "community event" which promoted trust and a good rapport with local health professionals. Thus, the intention that the organizers of Riverside's Health Fair had, of reaching-out to local residents was a fruitful endeavor for the entire community.

Discussion

The major objective of the Health Fair was to provide health care and social services for an African American community in a culturally-oriented and practical approach. After assessing the initial conceptualization of the health fair, the principal investigator recognized that there was a definite need to include a wider range of community services in the program. Information about services such as crime prevention, prenatal and child care counseling, AIDs education play, and free prizes/gifts/food from local radio and community businesses were provided not only as donations to an at risk population but also marketed and designed in a culturally-oriented approach. This culturally-oriented approach consisted of: (1) increasing the number of African American health care and social personnel; (2) promoting the event through traditional African American media; and (3) educating African Americans in a style and pattern of which they could understand and are accustomed to.

For example, advertising the community health screening through a combination of selected traditional African American medias (local churches, newspapers, markets, barbershops, radio stations, and community centers) was particularly important for the marketing of this event. In addition, services such as pre-natal counseling and the AIDs education play was written and presented specifically for an African American audience by a local African American performance group. Because of the familiarity and excellent rapport of the African American playwright and the community threatre group had already established with Houston's African American population, the AIDs play worked well. Thus, primary prevention efforts, such as this community health screening, must emerge from a knowledge of and a respect for the culture of the target community to ensure that both the community organization and development effort and any interventions that emerge are culturally-sensitive and linguistically appropriate (Bailey 1988 and LeMaile-Williams 1976).

CONCLUSION

This chapter has demonstrated how clinically-applied medical anthropologists are capable of fathoming the needs and peculiarities of major health care issues in the African American community. The culturally-oriented intervention strategies developed for the Houston and Detroit African American communities can be best summarized as:

1. involving individuals/group members in the planning process to maximize the likelihood that they will have an investment in the outcomes;

2. combining knowledge of sociocultural and psychosocial factors to produce the most favorable outcomes by targeting specific and known community needs and by not isolating physical health from overall community wellness.

3. using anthropological concepts and data to inform organizers more comprehensively about the cultural context, emphasizing aspects of which they had previously been unaware.

In our pluralistic health care system, experts unfortunately, do not perceive that understanding cultural patterns among various ethnic groups make a difference in patient care. This is precisely why clinically-applied medical anthropologists must continue to develop intervention strategies that are practical and multicultural for our expensive and ever-changing health care system.

Chapter 8

CONCLUSION

The major findings of this book yield the following information concerning urban African American health care: (1) specific reasons why African Americans utilized or avoided health screening services; (2) the pattern of health care seeking among the African American population; (3) the sociocultural and psychosocial factors that influenced their health care seeking pattern; and (4) the importance of understanding the concept of "culture" and the African Americans' health beliefs and practices as critical to health maintenance and prevention.

The qualitative data obtained during and after the 1986 Detroit health screenings and the 1989 Houston Health Fair form the basis of the findings of this study. The 27 individual health profiles, 176 semi-structured interviews and daily observations of Detroit and Houston African Americans provided the emic perspective about the lifestyles and health care seeking pattern. General and key informants indicated that "being healthy" encompasses a degree of activity and responsibility. Related to the informants definition of health were cultural values such as individual and family moral strength, an orientation to present time, and survival of the family. Since general and key informants had a broad definition of what constitutes "being healthy," they consequently had a different perception of what constitutes an "illness" as compared with that of health professionals.

Detroit African Americans' beliefs about the etiology of hypertension are based on primarily naturalistic agents. General and key informants considered inadequate rest, poor nutrition, weather disturbances, and imbalances in hot and cold properties as naturalistic agents affecting their blood pressure.

With regard to treatment actions for high blood pressure ("high blood"), informants were inclined to use home remedies and nonprescribed (patent) medicines suggested to them by their extended familial 'lay' network. General and key informants indicated that ethnotreatment for high blood pressure varied from altering one's activity to consuming such astringent substances as epsom salts, sassafras teas, garlic tablets, vinegar, lemon juice, aspirins, and cream of tartar. These substances were purchased from grocery stores as well as from alternative/folk health practitioners, such as herbalists and magic store vendors.

In most cases, informants used various ethnomedical treatment therapies prior to medical consultations and continued after consultation with the physician's prescribed medications, even though the informant did not tell the physician of this fact. Clearly, the inability of some informants to participate actively in the discussion of their illness affected not only the quality of care but also their adherence to prescribed treatment regimens.

In this study, I documented that certain West African ethnomedicine elements (including beliefs concerning health and the therapeutic practices of traditional folk healers) are still used among today's urban African Americans. To reiterate, the persistence of ethnomedicine provides a meaningful alternative to allopathic medicine for many African Americans because of its role in maintaining a sense of ethnic identity. Actually, major health care culture differences exist between ethnic groups in terms of health-related knowledge, attitudes toward health and therapeutics, health care seeking behavior, and the use of local health care facilities.

Ethnicity serves as a marker not just for supposed "folk" beliefs and practices, but for a broader range of beliefs and behaviors not usually labeled as "culturally different." Ethnic groups may experience different patterns of illnesses and may view certain symptom patterns as more salient than others. They may use different strategies in the home for managing illnesses and use different criteria for deciding to seek outside help. Their effective access to health care resources may be limited by language, by physical isolation, by social marginality and discrimination, and by recency of migration.

In view of the issues discussed in this book, there is an obvious need to focus on the cultural orientations of African Americans toward health care. Understanding the culture of an individual is of special importance in health-related situations, because it determines whether an individual will utilize or avoid available health care services. One's culture is a system of shared beliefs, values, customs, and behaviors that members of a society use in coping with one another and with their world, and that are transmitted from generation through learning. This learned culture guides health care action and health beliefs as the individual meets both familiar and new illness situations. Not only should health care professionals try to work "within" the cultural value system of the African

American patient, but also African Americans should attempt to work "with" the cultural value system of the health care professional. By doing this, both parties will benefit simply because of the powerful influences of cultural factors over a lifetime in shaping people's attitudes toward health behaviors and types of treatments. In addition, once more health care professionals and researchers begin to identify a "distinctive" preventative health care pattern among urban African Americans, critical health care issues such as the high prevalence of hypertension, cancers, diabetes, and infant mortality can be truly resolved.

REFERENCES CITED

Adair, John and Kurt Deuschle 1977 The People's Health. New York: Appleton-Century-Crofts.

Adams, Lucile et al. 1986 "Blood Pressure Determinants in a Middle-Class Black Population: The University of Pittsburgh Experience." Preventive Medicine 15:232-243.

American Heart Association 1983 High Blood Pressure. Dallas: American Heart Association's Office.

Aschenbrenner, Joyce 1973 "Extended Families Among Black Americans" Journal of Comparative Family Studies 4:257-268.

Baer, Hans 1985 "Toward a Systematic Typology of Black Folk Healers." Phylon 43:327-343.

Bailey, Eric 1988 "An Ethnomedical Analysis of Hypertension Among Detroit Afro-Americans" Journal of National Medical Association" 80:1105-1112.

1988 Hypertension: An Analysis of Detroit Afro-American Health Patterns. Dissertation Research. Wayne State University. Detroit, MI.

1987 "Sociocultural Factors and Health Care Seeking Behavior Among Black Americans" Journal of National Medical Association 79:389-392.

Bailey, Kenneth 1982 Methods of Social Research. 2nd Edition. New York: John Wiley and Sons.

Barnes, Annie 1981 "The Black Kinship System" Phylon 42:369-380.

Bauer, Gregory et al.   1983 "Effect of State and Trait Anxiety and Prestige of Model on Imitation." Psychological Reports 52: 375-382.

Becker, Marshal   1979 "Patient Perceptions and Compliance: Recent Studies of the Health Belief Model. In Compliance in Health Care, R.B. Haynes, ed. pp. 78-81. Baltimore: John Hopkins Press.

   1977 "The Health Belief Model and Prediction of Dietary Compliance: A Field Experiment." Journal of Health and Social Behavior 18:348-366.

   1975 "Sociobehavioral Determinants of Compliance with Health and Medical Care Recommendations." Medical Care 13:10-24.

Berry, Mary and John Blassingame   1982 Long Memory: The Black Experience in America. New York: Oxford University Press.

Billingsley, Andrew   1968 Black Families in White America. New Jersey: Prentice-Hall Inc.

Blendon, R. et al.   1989 "Access to Medical Care for Black and White Americans." Journal of American Medical Association 261:278-281.

Bloch, Bobbie   1976 "Nursing Interventions in Black Patient Care." In Black Awareness: Implications for Black Patient Care, Dorothy Luckraft, ed. pp. 27-35. New York: The American Nursing Company.

Boykin, Ulysses   1943 A Handbook of the Detroit Negro: A Preliminary Edition. Detroit: The Minority Study Associates.

Boyle, E.   1970   "Biological Patterns in Hypertension by Race, Sex, Body Weight, and Skin Color. Journal of American Medical Association 213:1637.

Braithwaite, R. and Lythcott, N.   1989   "Community Empowerment as a Strategy for Health Promotion for Black and Other Minority Populations" Journal of American Medical Association 261:282- 283.

Bullard, Robert   1989   In Search of the New South: The Black Urban Experience in the 1970s and 1980s. Tuscaloosa: The University of Alabama Press.

        1982   Blacks in the Sunbelt. Westport CT: Greenwood Press.

Byrne, D.G. and H.M. Whyte   1983   "State and Trait Anxiety Correlates of Illness Behavior in Survivors of Myocardial Infarction."   International Journal of Psychiatry in Medicine 13:1-9.

Caldwell, John R. et al.   1970   "The Dropout Problem in Anti-Hypertensive Therapy." Journal of Chronic Diseases 22:579-592.

Campbell, A.   1979   "Hypertension Control- A Categorial Approach to Comprehensive Health Promotion and Disease Prevention." In United States Department of Health and Human Services. Health Education & the Black Community. Washington, D.C.: U.S. Government Printing.

Cassel, John   1975   "Studies of Hypertension in Migrants." In Epidemiology and Control of Hypertension, Paul O., ed. pp 41. New York: Stratton Intercontinental.

Chino, Harriet and Lothar Vollweiler   1986 "Etiological Beliefs of Middle-Income Anglo- Americans Seeking Clinical Help." Human Organization 45:245-254.

Chrisman, Noel   1982   "Anthropology in Nursing: An Exploration of Adaptation." In Clinically Applied Anthropology: Anthropologists in Health Science Settings, Noel Chrisman and T. Maretzki, eds. pp. 117-140   Boston: D. Reidel Publishing.

       1977 "The Health Seeking Process: An Approach to the Natural History of Illness." Culture and Medical Psychiatry 1:351-377.

City of Houston Health and Human Services Department.   1987 The Health of Houston: Births, Deaths and Other   Selected Measures of Public Health 1984-1986. Houston.

Clark, Joette   1986 "Nutrition and Blood Pressure Control." Lecture Presented at Henry Ford Hospital (Detroit, Mi.) January 29.

Cockerham, William   1986   Medical Sociology. Englewood Cliffs, New Jersey: Prentice-Hall, Inc.

Comprehensive Health Planning Council of Southeastern Michigan 1981 Regional Profile 1980. Detroit:

Comstock, B.W.   1957 "An Epidemiologic Study of Blood Pressure Levels in a Biracial Community in the Southern United States. American Journal of Hygiene 65:271.

Crawford, Charles   1971   Health and Family: A Medical-Sociological Analysis. New York: The MacMillan Company.

Crosby et al. 1981 The African Experience in Community Development. Reynoldsburg, Ohio: Advocate Publishing Group.

Cruz-Coke, R. 1981 "Etiology of Essential Hypertension" Hypertension 3:191-194 (Supplement).

Cunningham, George 1972 Detroit. The Mayor and City Government: Learning About People, Places, and Things. Detroit: Elite Publishers Company.

Dawber, T.R. et al. 1967 "Environmental Factors in Hypertension" In The Epidemiology of Hypertension, J. Stamler, R. Stamler and T. Pullman, eds. pp. 255-288. New York: Grune and Stratton.

Deskins, Donald 1972 Residential Mobility of Negroes in Detroit. Ann Arbor: University of Michigan.

Detroit Urban League 1965 A Profile of the Detroit Negro: 1959-1964. Detroit: Research Department Committee.

Diamond, John 1967 "Comment" Detroit: Mayor's Committee for Human Resources Development.

Donnison, C.P. 1929 "Blood Pressure in the African Native" The Lancet 6-7.

Dressler, William 1984 "Social and Cultural Influences in Cardiovascular Disease: A Review" Transcultural Psychiatric Review" 21:5-42.

1982 Hypertension and Cultural Change: Acculturation and Disease in the West Indies. New York: Redgrave Publishing Company.

Elzy, Robert 1927 "Adjusting the Colored Migrant From the South to Life in a Northern City" Opportunity 175-176.

Erfurt, J. and Foote, A. 1984 "Cost-Effectiveness of Work-Site Blood Pressure Control Programs" Journal of Occupational Medicine 26:892-900.

Ewell, J. 1813 Planter's and Mariners' Medical Companion. Philadelphia.

Fabrega, Horacio 1975 "The Need for an Ethnomedical Science" Science 189: 969-975.

Feinstein, Otto 1974 "Why Ethnicity" In Immigrants and Migrants: The Detroit Ethnic Experience. David Hartman, ed. pp. 2-9. Detroit: New University Thought Publishing.

Fishwick, Marshall 1971 "Introduction" Black Popular Culture 3:637-645.

Fitzpatrick, John 1981 "Reflections on Being a Complete Participant" In Readings for Social Research. Theodore Wagenaar, ed. pp. 118-129. Belmont, CA: Wadsworth Publishing Company.

Franklin, John and Alfred Moss 1988 From Slavery to Freedom: A History of Negro Americans. New York: Alfred A. Knopf.

Garro, Lynda 1986 "Cultural Models of High Blood Pressure" Paper Presented at the 85th American Anthropological Association. Philadelphia, PA.

Geiger, H. 1972 "A Health Center in Mississippi: A Case Study in Social Medicine." In Medicine in a Changing Society. L. Corey, S. Saltman and M. Epstein, eds. St Louis: C.V. Mosby.

Goodson, Martia 1987 "Medical-Botanical Contributions of African Slave Women to American Medicine" The Western Journal of Black Studies 2:198-203.

Greater Detroit Area Health Council 1983 Health Care in Southeastern Michigan: An Assessment of the Environment. Detroit: GDAC.

Gutman, Herbert 1976 The Black Family in Slavery and Freedom. New York: Pantheon Books.

Haber, David 1986 "Health Promotion to Reduce Blood Pressure Level Among Older Blacks" The Gerontologist 26:119-121.

Hanna, J.M. and P.T. Baker 1979 "Biocultural Correlates to the Blood Pressure of Samoan Migrants in Hawaii" Human Biology 51: 481-497.

Harburg, Ernest et al. 1978 "Skin Color, Ethnicity, and Blood Pressure I: Detroit Blacks" American Journal of Public Health 68:1177-1183.

1973 "Socioecological Stressor Areas and Black-White Blood Pressure:Detroit" Journal of Chronic Disease 26:595-611.

1973 "Socioecological Stress, Suppressed Hostility, Skin Color, and Black-White Male Blood Pressure: Detroit" Psychosomatic Medicine 35:276-295.

Harding, Vincent 1981 There is a River: The Black Struggle for Freedom in America. New York: Vintage Books.

Harrison, Ira and Diana Harrison 1971 "The Black Family Experience and Health Behavior" In Health and the Family: A Medical-Sociological Analysis. Charles Crawford, ed. pp. 125-140. New York: The MacMillan Company.

Hartog, Joseph and Elizabeth Hartog 1983 "Cultural Aspects of Health and Illness Behavior in Hospitals" Western Journal of Medicine 139:910-916.

Harvey, William   1988 "Voodoo and Santeria: Traditional Healing Techniques in Haiti and Cuba" In Modern and Traditional Health Care in Developing Societies. Christine Zeichner, ed. pp. 101-114. New York: University Press of America.

Hays, W. et al.   1973 "Extended Kinship Relations in Black and White Families" Journal of Marriage and Family 35:51-57.

Haynes, M. Alfred   1975 "The Gap in Health Status Between Black and White Americans" In Textbook of Black-Related Disease. Richard Williams, ed. pp. 15-30. New York: Mc-Graw- Hill Book Company.

Henderson, George   1965 Aspirations and Social Class: An Analysis of Educational Obsolence. Unpublished Ph.D. Wayne State University.

Henry, James and John Cassel   1969 "Psychosocial Factors in Essential Hypertension" Journal of Epidemiology 90:171-197.

Herskovits, Melville   1941 The New World Negro. Bloomington, IN: Indiana University Press.

    1937 Life in a Haitian Valley. New York: Alfred Knopf Company.

Hill, Carole   1976 "Folk Medical Belief System in the American South: Some Pratical Considerations" Southern Medicine 11-17.

    1973 "Black Healing Practices in the Rural South" Journal of Popular Culture 6:849-853.

Hines, Paulette and Nancy Boyd-Franklin   1982 "Black Families" In Ethnicity and Family Therapy. M. McGoldrich and J. Pearce, eds. pp. 84-107. New York: The Guildford Press.

Hines, R.H.   1972   "The Health Staus of Black Americans: Changing Health Perspectives" In Patients, Physicians, and Illness. E.G. Jaco, ed. pp. 42-62. New York: The Free Press.

Hosten, Adrian   1980 "Hypertension in Black and Other Populations: Environmental Factors and Approaches to Management" Journal of National Medical Association 72:111-117.

Housing Authority of the City of Houston.   1983 Village/Fourth Ward. Allen Parkway Houston-Galveston Area Council Interagency Data Task Force.

    1983 Population and Employment Projections for Harris County: Regional Information Service.

Jackson, Jacquelyne   1985 "Race, National Origin, Ethnicity, and Aging" In Handbook of Aging and the Social Sciences. Robert Binstock and Ethel Shanas, eds. pp. 264-303. New York: Van Nostrand Publishing Company.

Jacques, Gladys   1976 "Cultural Health Traditions: A Black Perspective" In Providing Safe Nursing Care for Ethnic People of Color. Marie Branch and Phyllis Paxton, eds. pp. 115-123. New York: Appleton-Century Crofts.

Johnson, E.P. et al.   1983 "Induced Response Bias on the State-Trait Anxiety Inventory" Social Behavior and Personality 11: 113-117.

Johnson, E., Schork, N. and Spielberger, C.   1987 "Emotional and Familial Determinants of Elevated Blood Pressure in Black and White Adolescent Females" Journal of Psychosomatic Research 31: 731-741.

Joint National Committee on Detection, Evaluation, and Treatment of High Blood Pressure 1984 Arch. Internal Medicine 144:1045-1057.

Jones, E.   1986 "Preventing Disease and Promoting Health in the Minority Community" Journal of National Medical Association 78:18-20.

Jordan, Wilbert   1979   "The Roots and Practice of Voodoo Medicine in America" Urban Health 8:38-41.
    1975   Voodoo Medicine. In Textbook of Black-Related Diseases. Richard Williams, ed. pp. 716-738. New York: Mc-Graw-Hill Books Company.

Julius, S. and Johnson, E.   1985 "Stress, Autonomic Hyperactivity and Essential   Hypertension: An Enigma" Journal of Hypertension 3 (suppl 4):S11-S17.

Kaplan, Bernice   1988   "Migration and Disease" In Biological Aspects of Human Migration. Mascie-Taylor and G.W. Laker, eds. pp. 216-245. Cambridge: Cambridge University Press.

Katzman, David   1973   Before the Ghetto: Black Detroit in the 19th Century. Chicago: University of Illinois Press.

King, Jennifer   1982   "The Impact of Patient's Perceptions of High Blood Pressure on Attendance at Screening: An Extension of the Health Belief Model" Social Science and Medicine 16:1079-1091.

Kirscht, John   1974   "The Health Belief Model and Illness Behavior" Health Education Monographs 2:387-407.

Kleinman, Arthur   1980   Patients and Healers in the Context of Culture. Berkeley: University of California Press.

Kong, B. Wayne, Miller, Joseph, and Roland Smoot   1982 "Churches as High Blood Pressure Control Centers" Journal of National Medical Association 74:920-923.

Kornhauser, Arthur   1952   Attitudes of Detroit People Toward Detroit: Summary of Detailed Report. Detroit: Wayne State University.

Ladner, Joyce   1971   Tomorrow's Tomorrow. New York: Anchor Books.

Langford, H.G. et al.   1985   "Dietary Profile of Sodium, Potassium, and Calcium in United States' Blacks" In Hypertension in Blacks. W. Hall, E. Saunders and N. Shulman, eds. pp. 49-57. Chicago: Yearbook Medical Publishers Inc.

Langford, Herbert   1981   "Is Blood Pressure Different in Black People?" Postgraduate Medical Journal 57:749-754.

LaSater, Thomas et al.   1986   "The Role of Churches in Disease Prevention Research Studies" Public Health Reports 101: 125-131.

Lee, Alfred McClung   1943   Race Riot. New York: The Dryden Press.

Leininger, Madeleine   1985   "Southern Rural Black and White American Lifeways with Focus on Care and Health Phenomena" In Qualitative Research Methods in Nursing. Madeleine Leininger, ed. pp. 195-216. New York: Grune and Stratton.

        1985   Qualitative Research Methods in Nursing. New York: Grune and Stratton, Inc.

        1984   The Essence of Nursing and Health. New Jersey: Slack Inc.

LeMaile-Williams, Robert   1976   "The Clinical and Physiological Assessment of Black Patients" In Black Awareness: Implications for Black Patient Care. Dorothy Luckraft, ed. pp. 16-26. New York: The American Nursing Company.

Lewis, Eric   1985 "Personal Communication" Former Research Fellow. Endrocrinology and Metabolism Department at University of Michigan.

Lieban, Richard   1977 "The Field of Medical Anthropology" In Culture, Disease, and Healing: Studies in Medical Anthropology. David Landy, ed. pp. 13-30. New York: MacMillan Publishing Inc.

Lust, John   1974 The Herb Book. New York: Bantam Books.

Malec, Michael   1977 Essential Statistics for Social Research. New York: J.B. Lippincott Company.

Manuel, Ron   1986 "Demographics and the Black Elderly" Paper Presented at the 1986 Gerontological Meetings Chicago, Illinois.

Marks, Carole   1985 "Black Workers and the Great Migration North" Phylon 46:148-161.

Marmot, M.G.   1985 "Psychosocial Factors and Blood Pressure" Preventive Medicine 14:451-465.

  1985 "Psychosocial Factors and Blood Pressure" In Handbook of Hypertension. C.J. Bulpitt, ed. pp. 89-103. New York: Elsevier Science Publishers.

Mayer, Albert and Thomas Hoult   1962 Race and Residence in Detroit. Detroit: Institute for Urban Studies.

Mbiti, John   1975 Introduction to African Religion. Ibadan: Institute for Urban Studies.

McGhee, Ethel   1927 "The Northern Negro Family" Opportunity 176-178.

Mechanic, David   1980 "Health and Illness Behavior" In Public Health and   Preventive Medicine. John Last, ed. pp. 1035-1045. New York: Appleton-Century Crofts.

Miall, W.E. 1959 "Follow-Up Study of Arterial Pressure in Population of Welsh Mining Valley" British Medical Journal 2:1201-1210.

Miall, W.E. and P.D. Oldham 1963 "The Hereditary Factor in Arterial Blood Pressure" British Medical Journal 1:75-80.

Miall, W.E., Kass, E., and J. Ling 1962 "Factors Influencing Arterial Pressure in the General Population in Jamaica" British Medical Journal 2:497.

Michigan Metropolitan Information Center 1983 Michigan County Profiles: 1980 Census. Detroit: Center for Urban Studies, Wayne State University.

Miles, Norman 1978 Home at Last: Urbanization of Black Migrants in Detroit, 1916-1929. Ann Arbor: University of Michigan.

Miller, William 1986 "The Anthropology of Hypertension" Paper Presented at the 85th American Anthropological Association. Philadelphia, PA.

Mindel, Charles and Robert Habenstein 1981 "Family Lifestyles of America's Ethnic Minorities: An Introduction" In Ethnic Families in America: Patterns and Variations. Charles Mindel and Robert Habenstein, eds. pp. 1-13. New York: Elsevier.

Mittelmark, M. et al. 1986 "Community-wide Prevention of Cardiovascular Disease: Education Strategies of the Minnesota Heart Health Program" Preventive Medicine 15:1-17.

Morisky, Donald 1986 "Nonadherence to Medical Recommendations for Hypertensive Patients: Problems and Solutions" The Journal of Compliance in Health Care 1:5-20.

National Center for Health Statistics 1982 "Blood Pressure Levels and Hypertension in Persons Aged 6-74 years: United

States 1976-80" Advance Data from Vital Health Statistics DHHS Publication No. 82-1250.

Neighbors, Harold   1986   "Ambulatory Medical Care Among Adult Black Americans: The Hospital Emergency Room" Journal of National Medical Association 78:275-282.

New, Peter Kong-ming and New, Mary Louie   1977   "The Barefoot Doctors of China: Healers for All Seasons" In Culture, Disease, and Healing: Studies in Medical Anthropology. David Landy ed. pp. 503- 510. New York: MacMillan Publishing Inc.

Newmark, C.S.   1972   "Stability of State and Trait Anxiety" Psychological Reports 30:196-198.

Orgue, Modesta, Bloch, Bobbie and Lidia Monroy   1983   Ethnic Nursing Care: A Multicultural Approach. St. Louis: The C.V. Mosby Company.

Otten, M. et al.   1990   "The Effect of Known Risk Factors on the Excess Mortality of Black Adults in the United States" Journal of American Medical Association 263:845- 850.

Page, Lot   1980   "Hypertension and Atherosclerosis in Primitive and Acculturating Societies" In Hypertension Update. James Hunt ed.

    1974   "Antecedents of Cardiovascular Disease in Six Solomon Islands Societies" Circulation 49:1132.

Palmer, Dewey   1967   "Moving North: Migration of Negroes During World War I" Phylon 28:52-62.

Pinderhughes, Elaine   1982   "Afro-American Families and the Victim System" In Ethnicity and Family Therapy. M. McGoldrich and John Pearce, eds. pp. 108-122. New York: The Guilford Press.

Prineas, Ronald and Richard Gillum   1985   "United States Epidemiology of Hypertension in Blacks" In Hypertension in Blacks. W. Hall, Dallas Saunders, and N. Shulman, eds. pp. 75-110. Chicago: Yearbook Medical Publishers Inc.

Rabinowitz, Howard   1984   "A Comparative Perspective on Race Relations in Southern and Northern Cities, 1860-1900, with Special Emphasis on Raleigh" In Black Americans in North and South Carolina. Jeffrey Crow and Flora Hatley, eds. pp. 137-159. Chapel Hill: University of North Carolina Press.

Reilly, Joseph   1983   "Some Observations on the Recent Recession's Effects on the Detroit Area Health Care System" Urban Health 12:45-47.

Rogers, David et al.   1980   Health Care in the United States: Equitable for Whom. Beverly Hills, CA: Sage Publications.

Rubel, Arthur   1977   "The Epidemiology of a Folk Illness: Susto in   Hispanic America" In Culture, Disease, and Healing: Studies in Medical Anthropology. David Landy ed. pp. 119-128. New York: MacMillan Publishing Inc.

Runyon, Richard and Audrey Haber   1984   Fundamentals of Behavioral Statistics. London: Addison-Wesley Publishing Company.

Sampson, Calvin   1984   "Health Care Problems in the 1980's from a Black Perspective" Journal of National Medical Association 76:968-971.

Saunders, Elijah   1985   "Special Techniques for Management of Hypertension in Blacks" In Hypertension in Blacks. W. Hall and N. Shulman, eds. pp. 209-236. Chicago: Yearbook Medical Publishers Inc.

Scotch, Norman   1963 "Sociocultural Factors in the Epidemiology of Zulu Hypertension" American Journal of Public Health 53:1205-1213.

Scotch, Norman and H.J. Geiger   1963 "The Epidemiology of Essential Hypertension" Journal of Chronic Disease 16:1183-1213.

Sever, P.S. 1981 "Racial Differences in Blood Pressure: Genetic and Environmental Factors" Postgraduate Medicine 57: 755-759.

Shapiro, Alvin   1983 "Psychological and Social Factors in Hypertension" In Hypertension. Jacque Genesti, ed. pp. 765-775. New York: McGraw-Hill Book Company.

Shimkin, Demitri, Louie, G. and D. Frate   1978 "The Black Extended Family: A Basic Rural Institution and a Mechanism of Urban Adaptation" In The Extended Family in Black Societies. Demitri Shimkin, Edith Shimkin, and Dennis Frate, eds. pp. 25-147. Paris: Mouton Publishers.

Silver, George   1969 "What Has Been Learned About the Delivery of Health Care Services to the Ghetto" In Medicine in the Ghetto. John Norman, ed. pp. 71-90. New York: Appleton-Century Crofts.

Simic, Andrei   1985 "Ethnicity as a Resource for the Aged: An Anthro- pological Perspective" Journal of Applied Gerontology 4:65-71.

Sinclair, Robert and Bryan Thompson   1977 Metropolitan Detroit: An Anatomy of Social Change. Cambridge, Mass.: Ballinger Publishing Company.

Sing, Charles et al.   1986 "Genetics of Primary Hypertension" Clinical and Experimental Theory and Practice A8:623-651.

Snow, Loudell 1977 "Popular Medicine in a Black Neighborhood" In Ethnic Medicine in the Southwest. Edward Spicer, ed. Tucson, Arizona: The University of Arizona Press.
  1976 "High Blood is Not High Blood Pressure" Urban Health" 6:54-55.
  1974 "Folk Medical Beliefs and Their Implications for Care of Patients" Annals of Internal Medicine 81: 82-96.

Spector, Rachel 1979 Cultural Diversity in Health and Illness. New York: Appleton-Century Crofts.

Spielberger, Charles 1970 Manual for the State-Trait Anxiety Inventory. California: Consulting Psychologist Press.
  1960 Anxiety and Behavior. New York: Academic Press.

Spradley, James 1984 "Trouble in the Tank: Ethics in Urban Fieldwork" In Conformity and Conflict: Readings in Cultural Anthropology. James Spradley and David McCurdy, eds. pp. 52-66. Boston: Little, Brown, and Company.

SPSSx User's Guide 1983 New York: McGraw-Hill Book Company.

Thomas, James and James Dobbins 1986 "The Color Line and Social Distance in the Genesis of Essential Hypertension" Journal of National Medical Association 78:532-536.

Tinling, David 1967 "Voodoo, Root Work, and Medicine" Psychosomatic Medicine 29:483-490.

Turner, Arthur and Earl Moses 1924 Colored Detroit. Detroit: Burton Historical Collection of Detroit Public Library.

United States Bureau of Census 1988 Washington DC: U.S. Government Printing Office. 1982 Provisional Estimates of Social and Economic and Housing Characteristics. Washington D.C.: U.S. Government Printing Office.

1980 Washington DC: U.S. Government Printing Office.
United States Department of Health and Human Services   1986
   Black and Minority Health: Report of the   Secretary's Task
   Force: IV. Washington, DC: United States Government
   Printing Office.
Voors, A.W. et al.   1979 "Racial Differences in Blood Pressure
   Control" Science 204:1091-1094.
Wagenaar, Theodore   1981 Readings for Social Research. Bel-
   mont, CA: Wadsworth Publishing Company.
Warren, Donald   1975 Black Neighborhoods: An Assessment of
   Community Power. Ann Arbor: The University of Michigan
   Press.
Washington, Forrester   1920 The Negro in Detroit: A Survey of
   the Conditions of a Negro Group in a Northern Industrial
   Center During the War Prosperity Period. Detroit: Associated
   Charities of Detroit.
Weidman, H.   1982 "Research Strategies, Structual Alterations
   and Clinically Applied Anthropology. In Clinically Applied
   Anthropology: Anthropologist in Health Science Settings.
   Noel Chrisman and T. Maretzke, eds. pp. 201-241. Boston:
   D. Reidel Publishing.
Weissberg, P.L et al.   1987 "Genetic and Ethnic Influences on
   the Distribution of Sodium and Potassium in Normotensive
   and Hypertensive Subjects" Journal of Clinical Hypertension
   3:20-25.
Whitehead, T., Frate, D., Johnson, S.   1984 "Control of High
   Blood Pressure From Two Community Based Perspectives"
   Human Organization 43:163-167.

Wilkie, Jane   1976   "Urbanization and De-urbanization of the Black Population Before the Civil War" Demography 13: 311-328.

Williams, Roger et al.   1984   "The Genetic Epidemiology of Hypertension: A Review of Past Studies and Current Results for 948 Persons in 48 Utah Pedigrees" In Genetic Epidemiology of Coronary Heart Disease: Past, Present, and Future. D.C. Rao et al. eds. pp. 419-442. New York: Alan R. Liss Inc.

Wilson, P. et al.   1985   "Does Race Affect Hospital Use" American Journal of Public Health 75:263-269.

Wintz, C.   1984   "Blacks" In The Ethnic Groups of Houston. F. Melden, ed. pp. 9-40. Rice University Studies.

APPENDIX : Tables & Figures

TABLE 1.3: Estimated Population of Detroit: 1980

All Ages	Total	TOTAL Male	Female
	Total	Male	Female
All Ages	100.0	100.0	100.0
Under5	7.9	8.5	7.4
5-9	8.7	9.3	8.1
10-14	8.5	9.1	8.0
15-19	8.6	9.0	8.3
20-24	9.5	9.5	9.6
30-34	7.2	7.3	7.2
35-39	5.2	5.2	5.1
40-44	4.1	4.0	4.2
45-49	4.3	4.1	4.4
50-54	5.0	5.0	5.1
55-59	5.4	5.3	5.5
60-64	4.8	4.6	5.1
65&over	11.7	10.1	13.1
Under18	30.3	32.4	28.4

About 2.5 percent of total consists of persons
of race other than Black or White. Figures might
not add to 100.0 due to rounding.

TABLE 1.4: Estimated Population of Detroit: 1980

	Total	BLACK Male	Female
All Ages	100.0	100.0	100.0
Under5	8.9	9.6	8.3
5-9	10.4	11.2	9.7
10-14	10.2	11.0	9.6
15-19	9.7	10.1	9.3
20-24	9.4	9.1	9.7
25-29	8.9	8.4	9.4
30-34	7.6	7.2	7.9
35-39	5.6	5.4	5.7
40-44	4.4	4.1	4.6
45-49	4.4	4.1	4.6
50-54	4.8	4.7	4.6
55-59	4.6	4.6	4.6
60-64	3.7	3.6	3.7
65&over	7.5	6.8	8.2
Under18	35.6	37.7	33.6

TABLE 1.5: Estimated Population of Detroit: 1980

	Total	WHITE Male	Female
All Ages	100.0	100.0	100.0
Under5	5.8	6.3	5.4
5-9	5.3	5.8	4.9
10-14	5.4	5.8	5.0
15-19	6.6	6.9	6.4
20-24	9.7	10.1	9.3
25-29	9.0	10.1	8.1
30-34	6.6	7.3	5.9
35-39	4.4	4.8	4.1
40-44	3.7	3.9	3.6
45-49	4.0	4.0	4.0
50-54	5.6	5.6	5.6
55-59	7.0	6.6	7.3
60-64	7.2	6.7	7.7
65&over	19.7	16.3	22.8
Under18	20.3	21.8	18.9

About 2.5 percent of total consists of persons of race other than black or white. Figures might not add to 100.0 due to rounding.

(Comprehensive Health Planning of S.E. Mich 1981)

TABLE 1.6: Estimated Population of Detroit: 1980

TOTAL

	Total	Male	Female
All Ages	1,203,339	569,230	634,109
Under 18	364,618	184,394	180,224
Median Age	28.7	27.6	29.8
Dependency ratio	.72		

Totals include 30,670 persons of race other than black or white. Dependency ratio= population under 18 plus 65 & over divided by population 18-64 years old.

TABLE 1.7: Estimated Population of Detroit: 1980

BLACK

	Total	Male	Female
All Ages	758,939	355,676	403,263
Under 18	269,922	134,263	135,659
Median Age	25.8	24.5	26.8

Dependency
ratio   .76

TABLE 1.8: Estimated Population of Detroit: 1980

		WHITE	
	Total	Male	Female
All Ages	413,730	198,174	215,556
Under 18	83,861	43,199	40,662
Median Age	36.8	33.5	41.4
Dependency ratio	.66		

Totals include 30,670 persons of race other than black or white.

(Comprehensive Health Planning of S.E. Mich. 1981)

TABLE 1.9: Top Causes of Death in the State & Wayne County

Ranking	State	Wayne
1	Diseases of the Heart	Diseases of the Heart
2	Cerebrovascular Disease	Cerebrovascular Disease

3
Cancer of Respiratory
  Organs

Cancer of Respiratory
  Organs

4
Cancer of Digestive
  Organs

Cancer of Digestive
  Organs

5
Other Cancers

Other Cancers

6
Pulmonary Disorders

Homicide

7
Cancer of Genital
  Organs

Pulmonary Disorders

8
Motor Vehicle
  Accidents

Chronic Liver Disease

9

Other Accidents

Cancer of Genital
  Organs

Figure 3.2

Nonwhite Distribution in Detroit Metro Area

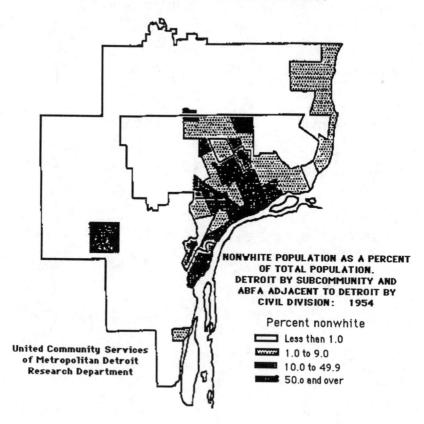

NONWHITE POPULATION AS A PERCENT
OF TOTAL POPULATION.
DETROIT BY SUBCOMMUNITY AND
ABFA ADJACENT TO DETROIT BY
CIVIL DIVISION: 1954

Percent nonwhite

Less than 1.0
1.0 to 9.0
10.0 to 49.9
50.0 and over

United Community Services
of Metropolitan Detroit
Research Department

(United Community Services of Detroit 1954:6)

Figure 4.1   HEALTH BELIEF MODEL

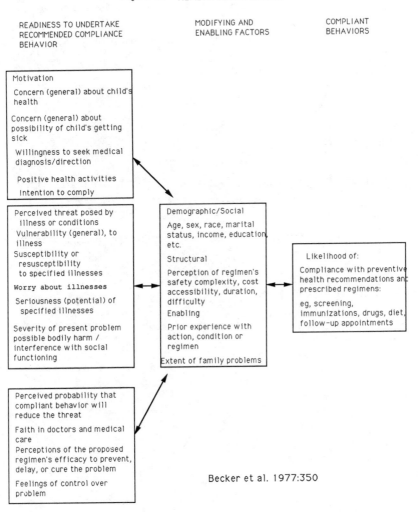

Becker et al. 1977:350

TABLE 5.4: Sex by Age and Ethnicity
Age Group (18 - 35 yrs.)

Sex	African Americans		Anglo Americans	
	N	(%)	N	(%)
Male	30	(61.2%)	4	(57.1%)
Female	19	(38.8%)	3	(42.9%)
	49		7	

Chi Square = 0.0, df = 1, p = 1.00

TABLE 5.5: Sex by Age Group and Ethnicity
Age Group (36 - 55 yrs.)

Sex	African Americans		Anglo Americans	
	N	(%)	N	(%)
Male	24	(34.8%)	3	(15.0%)
Female	45	(65.2%)	17	(85.0%)
	69		20	

Chi Square = 2.0, df = 1, p = 0.1

TABLE 5.6: Sex by Age Group and Ethnicity
Age Group (56 or older)

Sex	African Americans		Anglo Americans	
	N	(%)	N	(%)
Male	13	(23.6%)	17	(30.9%)
Female	42	(76.4%)	38	(69.1%)
	55		55	

Total =   173   Total =   82

Chi Square = 0.4, df = 1, p = 0.5
*Missing cases = 3

TABLE 5.7: Educational Level by Sex and
Ethnicity: Females

	African Americans		Anglo Americans	
	N	(%)	N	(%)
Less than 8 years	12	(11.7%)	4	(6.9%)
1-3HS	15	(14.6%)	7	(12.1%)
HS or Eqiv	43	(41.7%)	29	(50.0%)
Assoc.	11	(10.7%)	11	(19.0%)
B.A.	9	(8.7%)	4	(6.9%)
Grad.	13	(12.6%)	3	(5.2%)
	103		58	

Chi Square = 5.6, df = 5, p = .03

TABLE 5.8: Educational Level by

Sex and Ethnicity: Males

	African Americans N	(%)	Anglo Americans N	(%)
Less than 8 years	2	(2.9%)	2	(8.7%)
1-3HS	11	(16.2%)	1	(4.3%)
HS or Eqiv	41	(60.3%)	7	(30.4%)
Assoc	6	(8.8%)	6	(26.1%)
B.A.	6	(8.8%)	4	(17.4%)
Grad.	2	(2.9%)	3	(13.0%)
	68		23	

Total =   171   Total = 81

Chi Square = 14.2, df = 5, p =0.01
*Missing Cases = 6

TABLE 5.9: Educational Level by Age Group and Ethnicity
Age Group (18 - 35 yrs.)

	African Americans N	(%)	Anglo Americans N	(%)
Less than 8 years	1	(2.0%)	0	
1-3HS	5	(10.2%)	0	
HS or Eqiv	0	(61.2%)	2	(33.3%)
Assoc	10	(20.4%)	3	(50.0%)
B.A.	3	(6.1%)	1	(16.7%)
	49		6	

Chi Square = 4.2, df = 4, p = 0.3

TABLE 5.10: Educational Level by Age Group and Ethnicity
Age Group (36 - 55 yrs.)

	African Americans N	African Americans (%)	Anglo Americans N	Anglo Americans (%)
Less than 8 years	5	(7.1%)	0	
1-3HS	9	(12.9%)	1	(5.0%)
HS or Eqiv	34	(48.6%)	11	(55.0%)
Assoc	2	(2.9%)	3	(15.0%)
B.A.	9	(12.9%)	3	(15.0%)
Grad.	11	(15.7%)	2	(10.0%)
	70		20	

Chi Square = 6.9, df = 5, p = 0.2

TABLE 5.11: Educational Level by Age Group and Ethnicity
Age Group (56 or older)

	African Americans N	African Americans (%)	Anglo Americans N	Anglo Americans (%)
Less than 8 years	8	(14.8%)	6	(10.7%)
1-3HS	12	(22.2%)	7	(12.5%)
HS or Eqiv	22	(40.7%)	23	(41.1%)
Assoc	5	(9.3%)	12	(21.4%)
B.A.	3	(5.6%)	4	(7.1%)
Grad.	4	(7.4%)	4	(7.1%)
	54		56	

Total = 176   Total = 82

Chi Square = 4.6, df = 5, p = 0.4
*Missing Cases = 3

TABLE 5.12: Blood Pressure Distribution
African Americans

	Male		Female	
Systolic	N	(%)	N	(%)
80-139	41	(60.3%)	71	(67.6%)
140-159	20	(29.4%)	21	(20.0%)
160-240	7	(10.3%)	13	(12.4%)
	68		105	

Chi Square = 2.04, df = 2, p = 0.03

African Americans

	Male		Female	
Diastolic	N	(%)	N	(%)
60-89	42	(61.8%)	79	(75.2%)
90-114	26	(38.2%)	25	(23.8%)
115-130	0		1	(1.0%)
	68		105	

Chi Square = 4.6, df = 2, p = 0.09
*Missing Cases = 3

TABLE 5.13: Blood Pressure Distribution Anglo Americans

	Male N	Male (%)	Female N	Female (%)
Systolic				
80-139	15	(62.5%)	37	(63.8%)
140-159	7	(29.2%)	17	(29.3%)
160-240	2	(8.3%)	4	(6.9%)
	$\overline{24}$		$\overline{58}$	

Chi Square = 0.05, df = 2, p = 0.9

	Male N	Male (%)	Female N	Female (%)
Diastolic				
60-89	19	(79.2%)	42	(72.4%)
90-114	5	(20.8%)	16	(27.6%)
115-130	0		0	
	$\overline{24}$		$\overline{58}$	

Chi Square = 0.1, df = 1, p = .7

TABLE 5.14: Systolic BP by Age Group and Ethnicity
Age Group (18 - 35 yrs.)

	African Americans N	African Americans (%)	Anglo Americans N	Anglo Americans (%)
Systolic				
80-139	35	(70.0%)	6	(85.7%)
140-159	11	(22.0%)	1	(14.3%)
160-240	4	(8.0%)	0	
	$\overline{50}$		$\overline{7}$	

Chi Square = 0.9, df = 2, p = 0.6

TABLE 5.15: Systolic BP by Age Group and Ethnicity
Age Group (36 - 55 yrs.)

Systolic	African Americans		Anglo Americans	
	N	(%)	N	(%)
80-139	45	(64.3%)	17	(85.0%)
140-159	18	(25.7%)	2	(10.0%)
160-240	7	(10.0%)	1	(5.0%)
	70		20	

Chi Square = 3.1, df = 2, p = 0.2

TABLE 5.16: Systolic BP by Age Group and Ethnicity
Age Group (56 or older)

Systolic	African Americans		Anglo Americans	
	N	(%)	N	(%)
80-139	33	(60.0%)	30	(53.6%)
140-159	12	(21.8%)	21	(37.5%)
160-240	10	(18.2%)	4	(8.9%)
	55		55	

Total = 175   Total = 82

Chi Square = 4.2, df = 2, p = 0.1
*Missing Cases = 1

TABLE 5.17: Diastolic BP by Age Group and
Ethnicity
Age Group (18 - 35 yrs.)

Diastolic	African Americans		Anglo Americans	
	N	(%)	N	(%)
60-89	39	(78.0%)	6	(85.7%)
90-114	11	(22.0%)	1	(14.3%)
	50		7	

Chi Square = 0.0, df = 1, p =1.0

TABLE 5.18: Diastolic BP by Age Group
and Ethnicity
Age Group (36 - 55 yrs.)

Diastolic	African Americans		Anglo Americans	
	N	(%)	N	(%)
60-89	44	(62.9%)	14	(70.0%)
90-114	25	(35.7%)	6	(30.0%)
115-130	1		0	
	70		20	

Chi Square = 0.5, df = 2, p = 0.7

TABLE 5.19: Diastolic BP by Age Group
and Ethnicity

Age Group (56 or older)

Diastolic	African Americans		Anglo Americans	
	N	(%)	N	(%)
60-89	39	(70.9%)	42	(75.0%)
90-114	16	(29.1%)	13	(25.0%)
	55		55	

Total =   175   Total =   82

Chi Square = 0.07, df = 1, p = 0.7

TABLE 5.27: Multiple Regression for Systolic BP

Independent Variables	Beta	t	p=
Weight	-.05	-.89	.37
Sex	.04	.47	.63
Diagnosed Hypertensive	-.28	-4.26	.00*
Salted Food	-.06	-1.03	.30
Family History BP	-.00	-.08	.93
Ethnicity	.02	.27	.78
Education	-.16	-2.55	.01*
Perceived Symptom	-.16	-2.55	.01*
Unemployed	.17	2.70	.01*
Age	.13	2.06	.04*
Seek Physician	-.03	-.56	.57

```
Height              .17        1.74         .08
```

```
Multiple R = .49
R square   = .24
Stand. Error=.59
Adjusted R square = .21
```

*Significant Variables

TABLE 5.28: Multiple Regression for Diastolic BP

Independent Variables	Beta	t	p=
State Anxiety	.18	2.36	.01*
Weight	-.02	-.21	.82
Hypertensive	-.24	-3.55	.00*
Family History BP	-.13	-2.01	.04*
Salted Food	-.17	-2.64	.01*
Marital Status	.04	.49	.62
Ethnicity	.02	.26	.79
Perceived Symptom	-.08	-1.27	.20
Education	-.03	-.47	.63
Seek Physician	.04	.86	.39
Unemployed	-.01	-.20	.83
Height	.05	.48	.63
Age	.16	2.16	.03*
Sex	.07	-.68	.49

```
Multiple R = .51
R Square   = .26
Stand. Error=9.79
```

Adjusted R Square = .21

*Significant Variables